I0410617

Healthy Living Through Plant-Based Eating

Your Guide to Learning How to Move to Vegetarian/Vegan Eating

By Rod Stone

Table of Contents

Introduction

While the term "vegetarianism" is relatively knew, eating primarily a plant-based diet is not. In fact, many anthropologists believe early humans were more gatherers than hunters.

One fact supporting their views is that meat-eaters do not have molars as do humans. Another fact is that our digestive system more closely resembles other plant-eaters than it does meat-eaters. Third, relating to more recent times, humans that frequently eat meat are more of an increased risk for disease than their plant-eating colleagues drawing the conclusion humans were meant to eat plants and not animals.

Up until the mid-1900's, American ate more vegetables than meat. The meat consumed was done more on a local level due to the fact that without cold storage and efficient distribution yet, it was hard to get the meat to the people without it spoiling. To do so, meat had to be preserved in one of several methods which drove up the price and time to market.

The earliest vegetarian in recorded history was the Greek mathematician Pythagoras. In fact, early vegetarians were called Pythagoreans because word vegetarian had not been created yet. Other well-known names practicing eating primarily plants are Leonardo da Vinci, Benjamin Franklin, Albert Einstein and George Bernard Shaw. The term "vegetarian" was actually coined by the British Vegetarian

Society in the mid-1800's and comes from a Latin root word that means "source of life".

A vegetarian diet was first established in the United State with the 1971 release of Frances Moore Lappe's bestseller "Diet for a Small Planet". In her book she promoted more meatless meals in an effort to reduce the amount of resources it took to raise animals for food. At that time livestock were consuming 80% of the grain produced in the U.S. Her theory was that if America reduced meat consumption by 10%, there would be enough grain to feed the world.

However, vegetarianism was met with much speculation. The prevailing thought was it was impossible to get enough protein from eating just plant-based products. Through the rest of the 70's and well into the 80's, the myths prevailed until the release of John Robbin's book "Diet for a New America" in 1987. Part 2 of his book restarted the vegetarianism movement when he provided proof how dangerous animal diets were and conversely how safe plant-based ones were.

In the 1990's several documents were published highlighting the health value of plant-based diets including a paper by the American Dietetic Association endorsing the health benefits of vegetarian diets and the adoption of the Food Pyramid by the U.S. government. It showed Americans should eat mostly grains, fruits, vegetables, beans and less meat.

While a few of the myths are still around in limited numbers today, vegetarianism and the newer vegan diet have gained and continue to gain popularity and by all accounts are here to stay.

The truth is that we are all raised within a certain culture of food. And, for most people, this means that we are very used to eating meat. It can be quite daunting to think about completely giving it up forever, but at the same time it takes some time to adapt and get a real feel for a new diet. Especially if you have years of being a carnivore.

What is a Vegetarian Diet?

A vegetarian diet is one that excludes meat, chicken, and pork and mainly includes plant foods. There are various levels of exclusion of meat and animal byproducts, depending on the type of diet pursued by the individual. The reasons for following a vegetarian lifestyle vary, and include, health, ethical and religious justifications. Since the consumption of saturated fats that come from animal products has been linked with high cholesterol, and heart disease, many choose to eliminate those foods for health reasons alone.

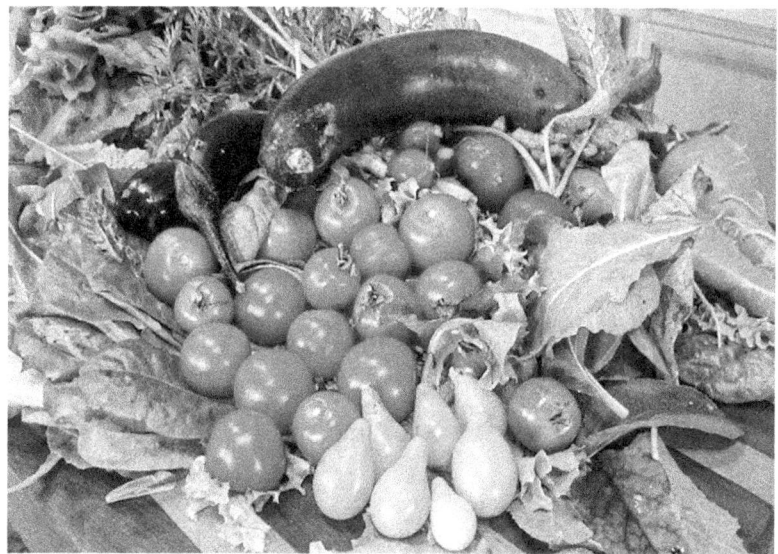

A plant-based diet focuses on vegetables, fruits, grains, nuts, and seeds. And oh boy there are so many different foods to choose from. You're going to be amazed at the variety. Many people feel like a plant-based diet is going to be restrictive. The opposite is true. When you come around to eating foods that are grown, rather than born, your mindset shifts and you realize the bounty that surrounds you.

Foods Omitted from A Vegetarian Diet:

The type of food omitted from a vegetarian diet depends on the specific type of vegetarian diet the person follows. In various forms, the following foods may be excluded:

- All animal products, including fish

- Eggs, milk, cheese and dairy

- Any non-food products made from animal or animal

  by-products

Vegetarianism in America

The use of plant diets is on the up rise. More and more people are choosing a meatless lifestyle or looking to get the bulk of their nutrition from plant foods.

✓ Almost 16 million Americans (5% of the population)

  are vegetarian and 50% of these people are vegan

  (Harris Interactive study commissioned by the

Vegetarian Resource Group). The number of vegetarians in the United States has doubled since 2009 when the count was only 2.5%.

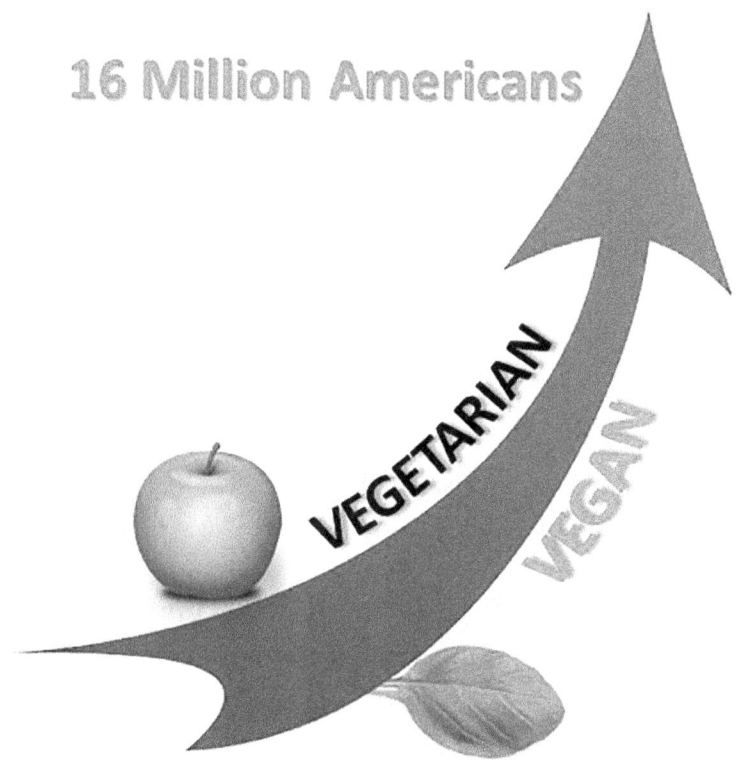

✓ Data also shows that 33% of Americans are eating vegetarian meals more often, even though they are not fully committed to the lifestyle.

✓ A 2010 Vegetarian Resource Group Nationwide poll found that 1.4 million people between ages 8 and 18 (3% of American youth) are vegetarian; this number is up from 2% counted 10 years ago.

What to Expect

It's often easier to stick with a lifestyle change, especially a major one, when you know what to expect. You can then make preparations to manage the challenges and look forward to the rewards. So let's explore what you can expect with a plant-based diet.

Withdrawal

Some people may experience a bit of withdrawal. It's not common, but when you completely eliminate something from your diet, your body can have a response. The most common side effect or withdrawal symptom is likely to be a little low energy or some digestive issues. Animal protein takes a lot of energy and time to digest. Plant-based protein and nutrients do not. You may experience more frequent trips to the bathroom. If you feel low energy or you are going to the bathroom too often, try adding some starchy vegetables to your diet. They can slow things down a little bit.

Cravings

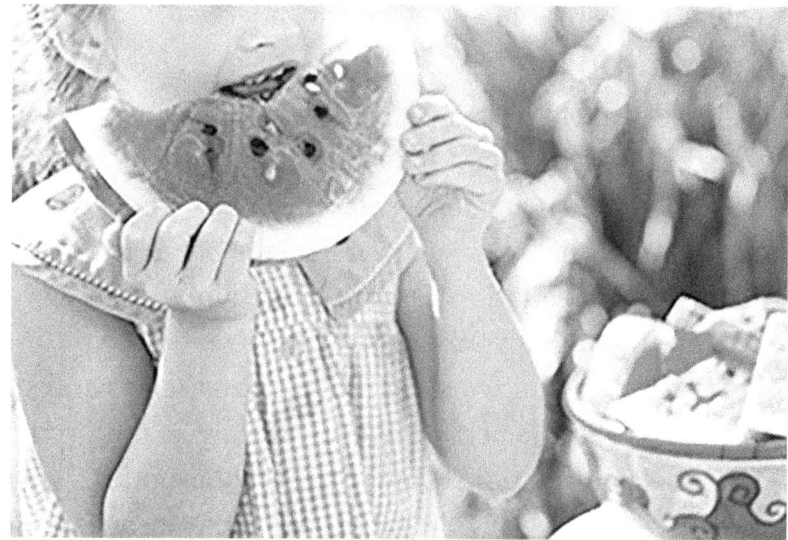

If you are a huge meat lover and your meals center on this food group, then you may have cravings. When you smell meat or see someone eating meat you may feel some urge to cave into your cravings. It's not common. Chances are you're going to feel so awesome and you'll be eating so well that you won't care.

However, if you do have cravings then find a food that you love and keep it with you. When you have cravings you can turn to your favorite food. For example, avocados are a treat. Spread half of one on a piece of whole wheat toast, sprinkle a little salt on it and enjoy.

More Planning

One of the biggest adjustments from a plant-based diet is the meal planning that's initially required. You're shifting to meals and food groups that you're not used to. After a week or two of eating this way, you'll find that meal planning is no longer a problem. Get a great cookbook or find a good vegetarian recipe blog to support you.

Explanations

Some people just won't understand why you're not eating meat and you can expect a lot of questions about your choice. Decide, in advance, what questions you're willing to answer and what your answers might be. You don't owe anyone an explanation, and you certainly don't have to convince them that your way is right.

However, if you focus on the positive aspects and share how diverse and delicious your diet really is, then you may enjoy the conversations. One common question is, "is there anything you can eat?" Which of course the answer is, "I can eat everything that you eat with the exception of animals. My diet is varied, delicious, and nutritious."

Rewards

You're probably already familiar with the benefits of a plant-based diet. It's why you've chosen this challenge. As a quick refresher, the rewards for a plant-based diet include but certainly aren't limited to:

- More Energy
- Better Sleep
- Improved Health (And Skin)
- Weight loss

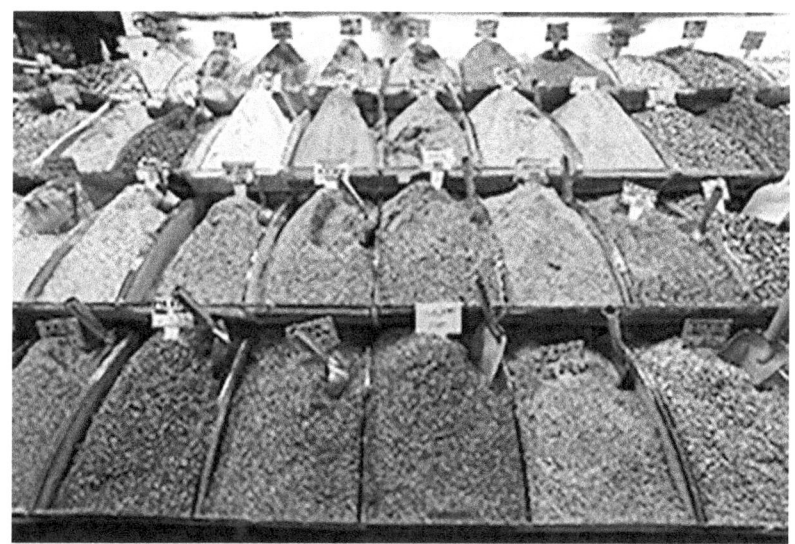

30 Tips for Success

Okay, so you have your plan in place. You know what approach you're going to take. You have your knowledge base of plant-based foods. You know what to expect and you're ready to get started. Awesome! Here are 10 tips to help you have the best 30-day challenge.

Tip #1 – Clean it out

Clean it out. Grab a basket and clean out your kitchen. Clean out your pantry, cupboards, refrigerator, and freezer. Get rid of all of your animal products. If you feel like this is wasteful, there are a few approaches. You can donate the food to a friend or family member. You can also ask a friend or family member to store it for you. If you're only doing a 30-day challenge, then this will work. If you're considering making it a lifestyle change, then donate the food.

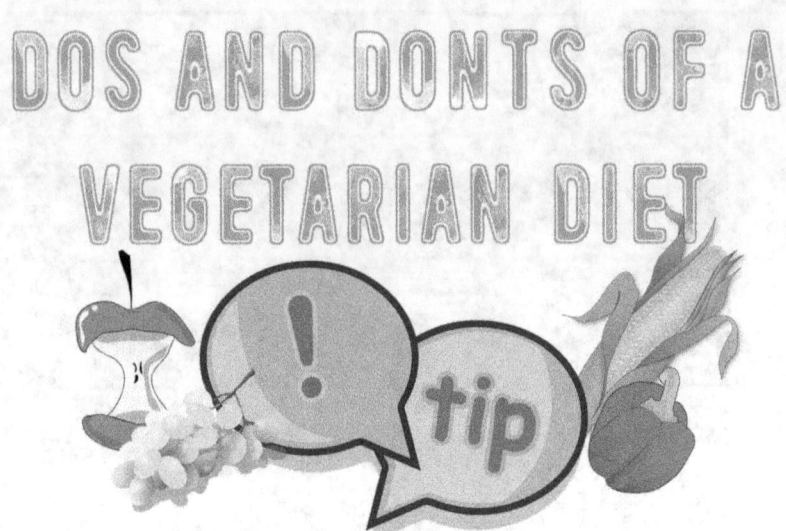

Tip #2 - Start Off with Meatless Mondays

Eliminating meat is not something you want to do cold turkey. You should slowly work your way into an all-meatless diet. You can do this by starting with Meatless Mondays. Eliminating meat from just one meal a week is a great way to test out and ease into this new lifestyle. Most dishes can easily be made vegetarian. For example, if pizza is one of your favorite foods you can remove the meat and pile on as many vegetables as you want or use tofu sausage. The key is to start small so you won't overwhelm yourself. If you try to do too much too soon you will be less likely to stick with this new way of eating. Even if you decide going meatless is not ideal for you, incorporating even one or two meatless meals a week can go a long way to better health.

Tip #3 - Make Sure You Vary Your Diet

There are many different plant foods to choose from, and contrary to what some may believe vegetarians do not just eat lettuce all day long. There are hundreds of imaginative and tasty recipes for vegans, many of which simply replace meat in old time favorite dishes. The sky is the limit and that is a good thing because like any other healthy eating plan it is important to eat a wide variety of different foods each day to be sure to get all the nutrients the body needs.

Tip #4 – Stand Strong

Not everybody will embrace your new lifestyle, and some friends and even family members may even mock you or poke fun. This happens to many people. Change is scary, but you must stay strong! Connect with other vegans and vegetarians for support. There are many online forums and discussion boards dedicated to living a vegetarian lifestyle where you can find likeminded people.

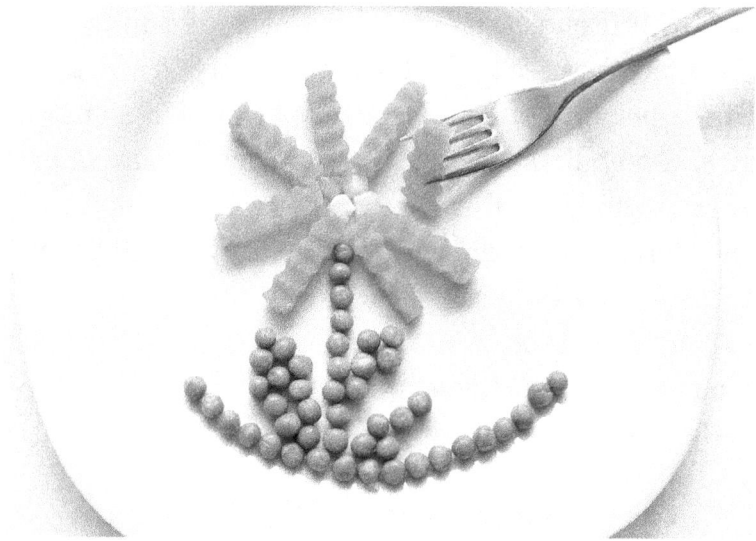

Tip #5 – Make It Fun!

If you are newly starting this lifestyle and have older kids, make the transition fun and easy for them by creating games and excitement around vegetarian living. Plant a garden with the kids, where each child chooses something to plant. Have each child choose their own signature vegetable or fruit and create special events, like cookouts around it each weekend. Make fun smoothies and have kids help with chopping of the fruit and preparation. Many fun vegetables recipes online will make this transition more exciting for the kids.

Tip #6 - Have A Family Recipe Challenge

Eating meatless is not easy, especially if you are used to eating meat with every meal so to make the process fun consider having a family recipe challenge. This can also be done with friends. The idea is for each person to come up with a meatless recipe for the others to try.

The person with the best recipe can win some sort of prize. Generally speaking, bragging rights may often be a reward in itself. Do this once a month or even once a week if time allows and by the end of the year, you will have many meatless dishes you can use regularly.

Find a good source of vegetarian recipes. You might buy or borrow a book. Blogs and vegetarian websites are also good resources.

Tip #7– Meal Planning

Meal planning. Plan your meals ahead of time and shop by your plan. This way you won't get stuck at a fast food drive through where your only plant option is French fries.

Tip #8 - Don't Be Afraid to Be Adventurous

To go meatless requires a certain level of adventure. You can't be afraid to try new things. There are so many recipes from different cultures that can be made without meat. You need to be willing to try as many as possible. Bring Turkey, Italy, Asia, and Greece into your kitchen. You will be surprised how much you enjoy trying meatless dishes from different cultures.

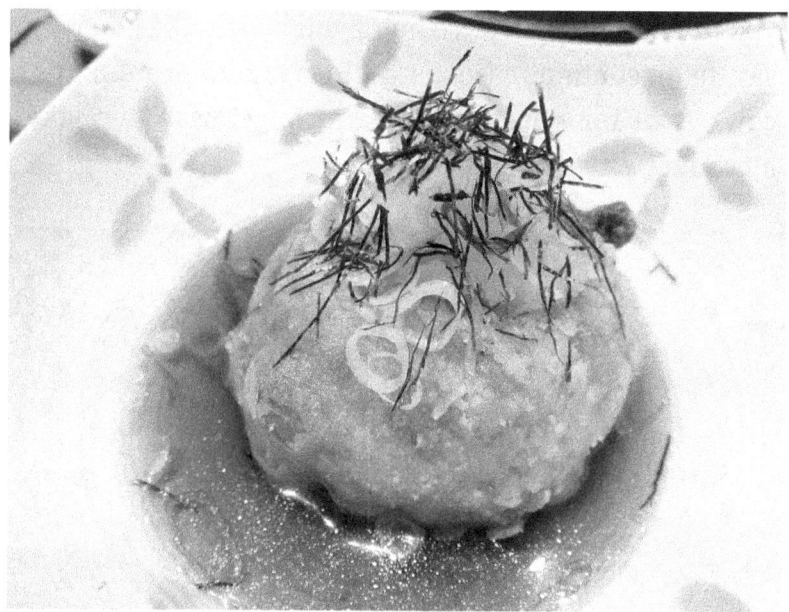

Tip #9 - Experiment! Experiment! Experiment!

To make your new lifestyle a success, it's important to experiment with different meatless dishes. If you aren't quite ready to make a meatless meal at home, consider trying one out at your favorite restaurant. This way you can get ideas of what you do and do not like.

Explore. Go to the supermarket and explore your options. Peruse all of the nuts, seeds, veggies, fruits, whole grains and meat and dairy alternatives. Get to know your food groups. If you see a food you're curious about, buy it and give it a try.

Tip #10 – Learn to read labels.

Learn to read labels. We already talked about the fact that some products contain animal products. For example, you might buy soy cheese but if you look at the label it might say that it contains casein. Casein is a dairy protein. It's from cows. Look for words "vegan" and "vegetarian" to make sure a product is truly plant-based.

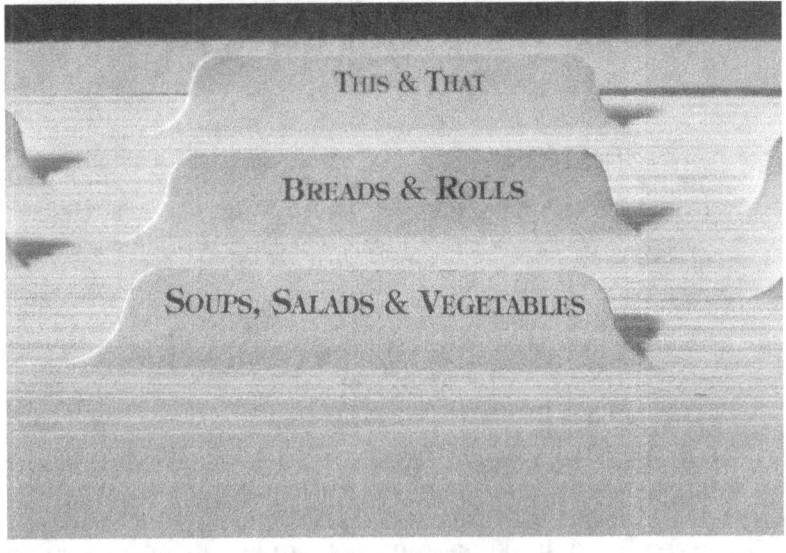

Tip #11 – Start A Recipe Collection

In order for anyone to stick with a certain way of eating, the menu must be well planned, diverse, and interesting. Starting a vegetarian or vegan recipe collection is a great way to ensure that you have access to tasty and diverse dishes that will prevent boredom and increase the chances of sticking with a meatless lifestyle.

Tip #12 - Don't Be Afraid to Have a Cookout

As a new vegetarian, you may think you can't enjoy a cookout with the family due to limited food options. This is completely false. You can get out there and barbecue with everyone else, the key is to plan. While you can't have a grilled chicken breast or a slab of ribs, you can enjoy soy burgers, soy hot dogs, fruit kabobs, all types of salads, grilled veggies, and potatoes.

Tip #13 - Make Sure You Get Plenty of Protein

One of the issues people run into when changing over to a meatless diet is not getting enough protein. It is important to get into the practice of reaching for plant sources of protein. If you don't get enough protein in your diet you will not feel satisfied and your health may suffer as the amino acids provided by protein play a crucial role in bodily functions. As a result, you may abandon meatless meals altogether.

Plant based sources of protein are plentiful, and you should make the effort to try as many as possible to find those you love. Learn to make proper meat substitutions in your favorite recipes, such as replacing meat with black beans in chili and tacos or using chickpeas to make meatballs for pasta. Use tofu in stir-fry, stews, and soup.

Snack on nuts and seeds and add half an avocado to your lunch plate.

Tip #14 – Learn to Substitute

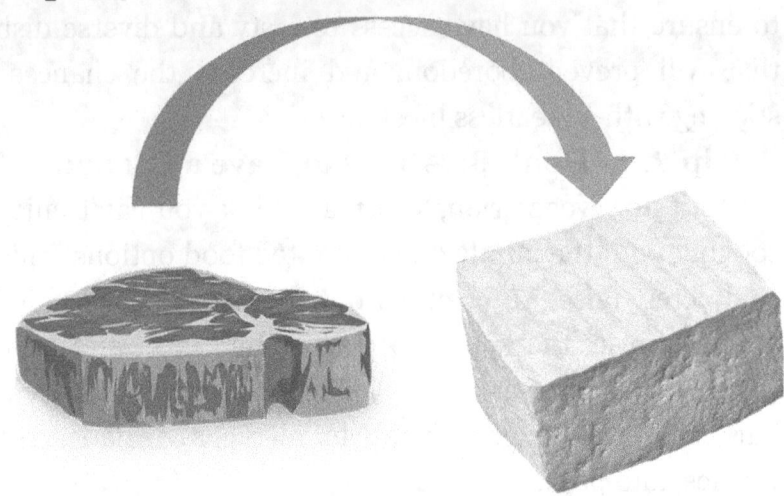

As a vegetarian, you will eliminate meat from your diet. As a result, you will have to figure out new ways to get all the nutrients you need on a regular basis and to learn to make appropriate substitutions so you can still enjoy your favorite dishes. Many of your favorites that include meat can be made vegan. For breakfast, try soy sausage patties and make chickpea patties or vegetable lasagna for dinner.

In the beginning, this may seem like a difficult task, but with experience and learning you will soon know exactly what to reach for in preparing the dishes you love without meat and chicken.

Tip #15 – Herbs and spices

Herbs and spices keep it interesting. If you love flavor, then you'll have fun using spices and herbs with your vegetarian dishes. For example, a little blend of pistachios, olive oil, and garlic is delicious. There are dozens of herbs and hundreds of spices to consider trying.

Tip #16 - Keep Nuts Around

Nuts make the perfect vegetarian snack. Just make sure you choose the unsalted and unflavored varieties. They taste great and provide a ton of health benefits. Besides snacking on nuts, they can replace cheese and meat in salads and add a crunchy topping to steamed vegetables. Natural trail mix is also a great snack.

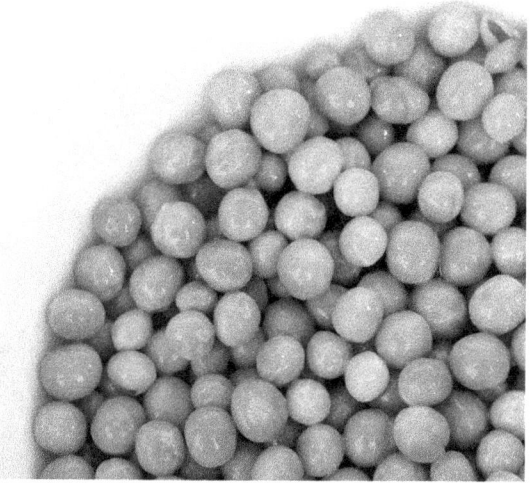

Tip #17 - Fill Up On Beans & Peas

Beans and peas are both high quality proteins that are very low in fat. Beans are also great sources of fiber. Because of this, it is recommended that vegetarians consume both foods on a regular basis. You can have a three-bean salad, bean tacos, chickpea burgers or falafel, pea soup, or vegetarian chili, just to name a few.

Tip #18 - Try New Fruits and Vegetables

You would be surprised how many fruits and vegetables are available and what you can do with them. Many vegetarian meals look and taste just as good, if not better, then the non-vegetarian option. The big difference however is they are a lot healthier for you.

Try new fruits and vegetables, you will likely find some that you have never tasted before. Make smoothies and homemade vegetable juices for refreshing and healthy meals and snacks. Try different cooking methods and recipes for vegetables and consume them in raw form on a regular basis.

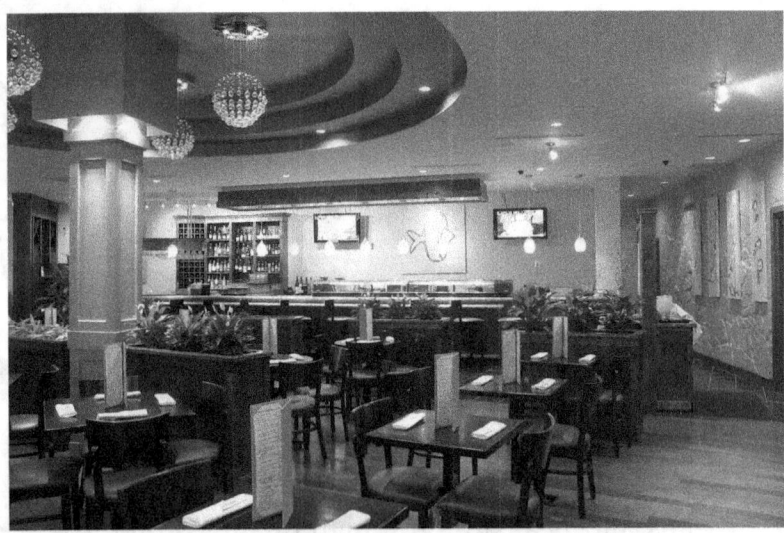

Tip #19 – Eating out

When eating out... eating out can be a challenge. The best thing that you can do is go prepared. Check out the menu before you go to a restaurant to make sure they have vegan and vegetarian options. Keep in mind that salads and salad dressings are an option. Pasta can be as well (if you eat eggs).

And don't hesitate to ask your waiter or server about ingredients and options.

Just because you are a vegetarian doesn't mean you can't go out to your favorite restaurant and enjoy a meal. The key is learning how to make the right substitutions. Most restaurants will gladly make vegetarian modifications for their guests. All you have to do is ask. Some restaurants offer soy options to substitute meat, soy cheese as a substitute for regular cheese, gourmet salads, and veggie burgers. If you live in a metropolitan area, there are usually plenty of vegan cafes where the entire menu is meatless. Before heading out to a restaurant go online and do a little research by looking at menus.

Tip #20 – Take A Vegetarian Cooking Class

How fun is that idea? Not only will you learn to cook vegetarian dishes you can meet and network with likeminded people.

Tip #21 – Variety

Variety. If you are someone who enjoys eating a lot of different foods, then embracing variety will be important. Keep in mind that the list of grains, veggies, fruits, nuts and so on that we've provided are just a portion of what's out there for you to try.

Tip #22 – Limit Sweets and Junk Food

Please realize that just because you stop eating meat, it does not mean you are consuming a diet low in saturated fat and cholesterol when it includes too many sweets, and junk food.

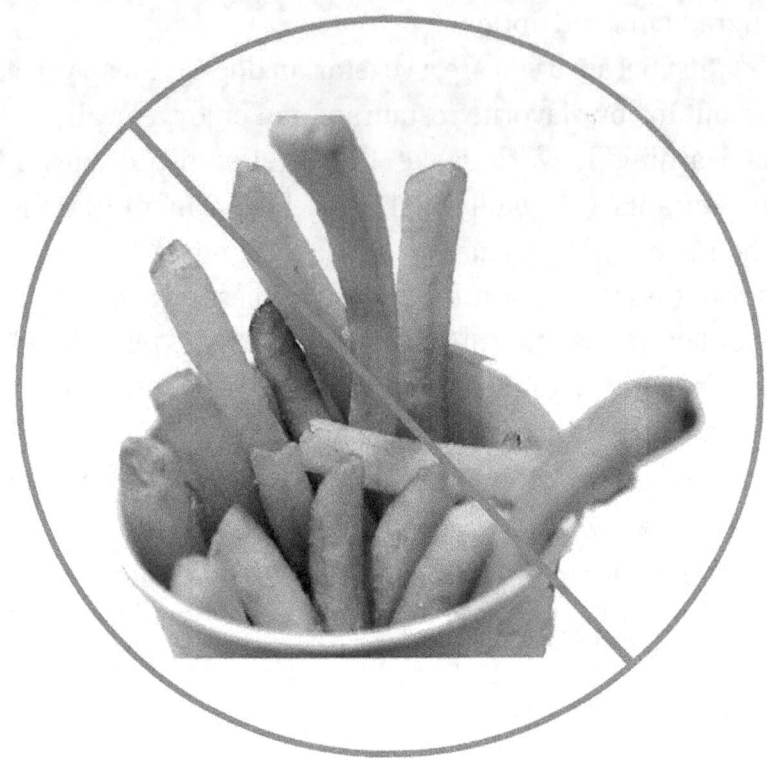

Becoming a vegetarian does not shield you entirely from unhealthy eating and the maze of junk foods available in our society. Meatless diets, like any others are about making healthy choices. French fries, donuts, candy, ice cream, white bread, pies, cakes, cookies and potato chips are all vegetarian, but not healthy and especially in large amounts.

Vegetarian snacks are also becoming easier to find as many people switch to this healthier lifestyle. However, not all of these are healthy options. Junk food is junk food and just because it is vegetarian doesn't mean that it's good for you. Moderation is key, be sure to treat yourself, but don't allow one of these delicious treats to become your regular go to snacks.

Keep in mind that to reap the health benefits, a vegetarian,
and vegan diet should consist primarily of plant foods.

Some people go haywire on cookies and cake because they think that their vegetarian diet compensates for all other poor nutritional choices, but this is simply not true. Not only does junk food and sweets pack on the weight, they are typically loaded with heart health unfriendly saturated fats.

Tip #23 – Don't be a junk food vegetarian

Don't be a junk food vegetarian. You probably know the vegetarian   who gained weight when they went meat-free. This is likely because they're getting their calories from starchy carbohydrates.

Sure, potato chips are plant-based but… they're certainly not nutritious. As a vegetarian it's important to make sure you're getting your nutrients. This is particularly important for B vitamins and protein requirements. Consider taking a protein supplement as well as a B complex vitamin.

Tip #24 – Don't Compare Everything to Meat

Some get into the habit of comparing all the soy substitutes to meat, like veggie burgers or soy hot dogs or chicken nuggets. This is a typical pitfall. Learn to appreciate all the new and distinct flavors.

Tip #25 - Appreciate The Health Benefits

If you have a high A1C, (type 2 diabetes) or high cholesterol, check the numbers again after 6 months.

Tip #26 – Be Kind to Yourself

If you slip and have a steak, it's okay, forgive yourself and start again.

Tip #27 – Eat In-Season Produce

Shop by seasonal produce. Seasonal fruits and veggies taste best when they're in season. If you're unsure what's in season this US government page has a brief overview: https://snaped.fns.usda.gov/nutrition-through-seasons/seasonal-produce.

This way you save money and the produce tastes much better.

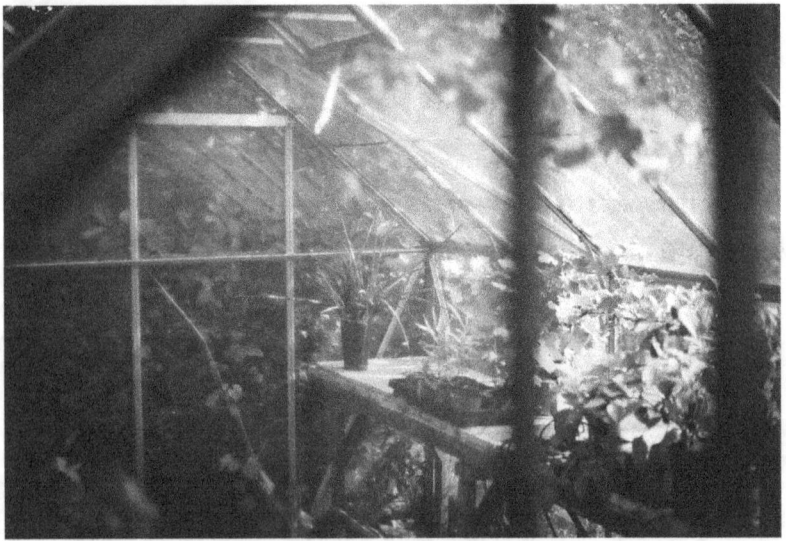

Tip #28 – Plant an Organic Garden

Fresh, no pesticides and within easy reach, enough said!

Tip #29 – Figure Out What You Will Do with All That Extra Energy

Plant foods provide so much energy that you will need to make a list of how you will use it!

Tip #30 - Find A Vegetarian Pattern That Works for You

No two vegetarians are alike. You have to find a plan that works best for you. Changing over to an all-vegetarian diet is not easy. That's why it is so important you take your time and find your own way. Follow the tips listed above and your transition will be a lot smoother.

Raising Vegetarian/Vegan Children

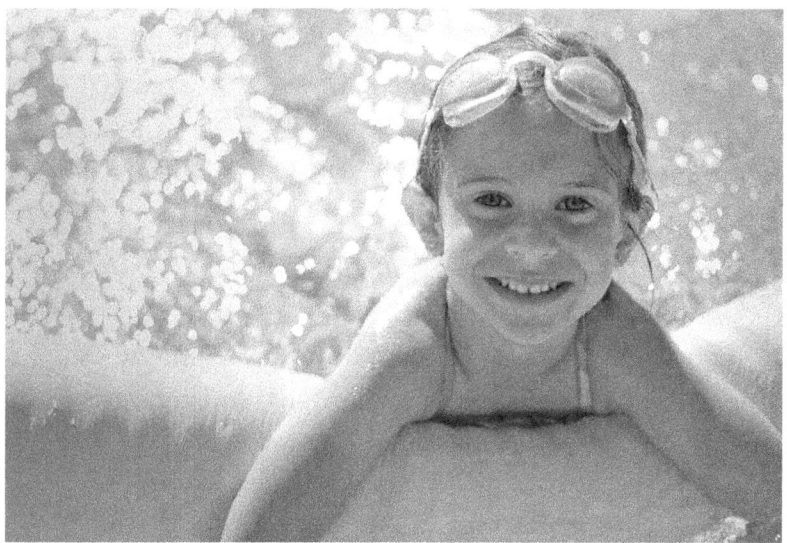

Nutritious vegan and vegetarian diets are typically high in fiber, full of antioxidants, vitamins, and minerals. They are also inherently low in saturated fat, rich in healthy plant protein and completely free of cholesterol.

Dr. Jatinder Bhatia, chairman of the American Academy of Pediatrics' committee on nutrition states that vegetarian diets for kids can be healthy as a long what is omitted is balanced with appropriate substitutes.

One of the more common concerns for vegetarian kids, as it is for adults is iron deficiency, because iron is more difficult to absorb from plant foods. This is why it is important to notify the pediatrician that the child is not eating meat so they can test for iron deficiency. This is most important because such a deficiency may not become apparent until the child is older, and at that point, there may be irreversible cognitive defects.

Kids raised on a lacto-ovo vegetarian diet eat dairy and eggs are at the least risk for under nutrition. The vegan diet is most restrictive and poses risks for B12, vitamin D, calcium, zinc, protein and riboflavin deficiencies, and it is most important that those nutritional needs are addressed appropriately.

According to Rebeca Roach, a registered dietitian and teaching associate at the University of Illinois' Department of Food Science and Human Nutrition comments while it is very difficult to raise a vegan child, it can be done as long as the parent completely understands their child's nutritional needs.

It is also important to note that unlike adults, a child's needs of particular nutrients will change through the developmental years, and those needs should be considered.

Parents who do not possess such understanding need to get the proper education. This can be obtained from books, authority sources online, or better yet a registered dietician and they need to communicate regularly with the pediatrician.

Two of the most common mistakes that parents make are to overcompensate for protein by feeding their kids an undue amount of foods high in saturated fat and calories, and the other is simply removing the meat without adding an appropriate replacement.

Exposing kids to a variety of different foods in various colors, textures and flavors develops a diverse palette as they age, provides optimal nutrition, and teaches them to be comfortable eating and trying a variety of different foods.

Modern Convenience

The good news is that it is much easier these days to raise vegetarian and vegan kids since meatless diets have become so widespread and therefore a variety of vegan and vegetarian foods are readily available at most any supermarket, including, soymilk, tofu, an array of fresh produce, and various vegan ready-made foods.

The Power of the Lunch Box

Do you remember when you were a kid how the idea of eating your vegetables made you desire a Big Mac sandwich even more? Well, that kind of reaction is fading fast as mothers promote the idea of eating vegan or vegetarian to their children and get creative while doing so. Today, you can refer to a number of meatless recipes online that are both vegan-and-kid-friendly at the same time.

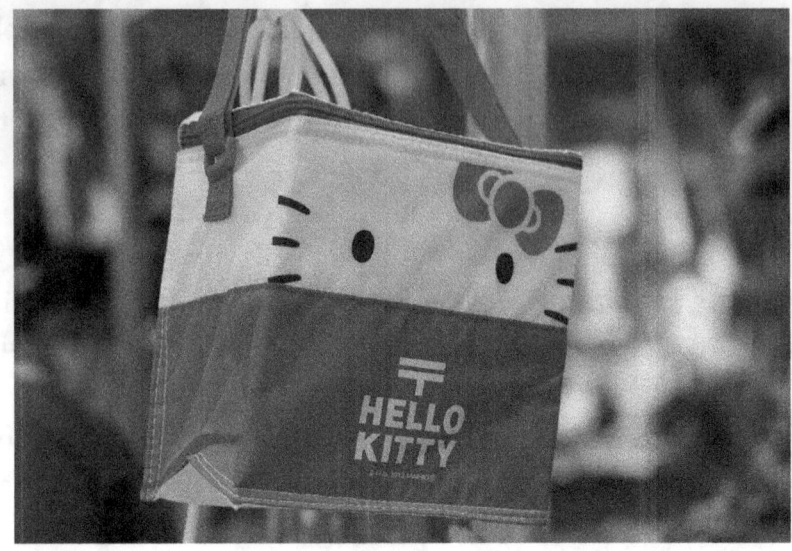

It is important to notify your pediatrician that your child is vegetarian so they can monitor for nutrient deficiency. Replace meat protein with plant sources. Make sure to include plant foods rich in iron, B12, calcium, riboflavin, and zinc to meet their growing needs.

One way to incorporate the idea of vegetarian and vegan foods into your kid's life is by including a wide variety of types of foods into their lunch box.

Incorporate Variety

To incorporate variety, vary the kinds of breads that you use for your kid's sandwiches. Use such breads as whole grain rolls, pita pockets, bagels, tortillas, or raisin bread to keep your child's interest from waning with respect to healthy eating.

You also want to make your child's thermos fare a treat. How about vegan macaroni and cheese, soup or leftover casserole to please their taste buds? If your child can microwave the meal at school, he can repurpose the food into a lunch entree.

Fruit Selections

Needless to say, lunch box fruits can come in an array of colorful offerings. Try adding small bits of fruits on a skewer or long cocktail toothpicks. Fruits such as grapes, melons, strawberries, apples and orange sections are always well received. If you include apples or pear slices, add small container of peanut butter for dipping in your kid's lunch box as well.

Veggies That Go with Dips

What holds true with peanut butter and fruit also holds true with respect to raw veggies and dips. If you include carrots, for instance, in your child's lunchbox, you can also add wedges of pita bread and a hummus dip. Besides carrots, veggies that go well with dips include bell peppers, and celery.

Turn Your Kid's Lunch into Brunch

Breakfast cereal can also be served in a lidded lunch bowl container and included with a non-dairy milk, such as vanilla almond milk, and a banana. Muffins are good substitutes for sandwiches. You can find recipes for such muffin specialties as zucchini and raisin muffins or blueberry muffins online. Include some soy cheese, fresh fruit, or soy yogurt with the muffin.

Salads with Kid Appeal

Salads that are included in wraps or pita bread will always appeal to the vegan kid who wants to experience a bit of adventure while eating. Add simple lettuce salads that feature veggie goodies like cucumbers, peppers, tomatoes, chickpeas, baked tofu, and grated cheese. Tofu can be used as a chicken replacement in chicken salad. Add pasta salad for an appealing lunch entrée. Again, diversity is the key. Include such shapes as elbows, wagon wheels, and shells. Combine the pasta with such veggies as broccoli, peas, carrots, and corn. Round out the lunchtime fare with a favorite salad dressing or soy yogurt topping.

Faux Turkey and Burger Cuisine

While we know that kids typically like peanut butter, you may also try including nut butters that feature sunflower, almond or cashew spreads. A warmed veggie burger placed on an English muffin or whole grain roll is a good lunch "sandwich" to include for a teen or older child. Faux turkey or chicken meats are appreciated as well in lunchtime vegan meals.

Diversity is the Key that Unlocks the Door to Vegetarian or Vegan Meal Planning

For dessert, add such vegan goodies as rice cakes, applesauce, fruit cups, graham crackers, bag of raw unflavored nuts or granola bars.

Note: It is advisable to not add any unusual or "weird" vegan foods as ridicule from other kids can quickly sour the whole vegetarian idea for your kids.

Types of Vegetarian Diets

Not all who call themselves "vegetarians" will eat the same things. There are different levels of vegetarianism that dictate what the individual can and cannot eat; here are the main types and the foods they include

There are seven different forms of vegetarianism and each one has its own set of parameters.

Vegan Diet

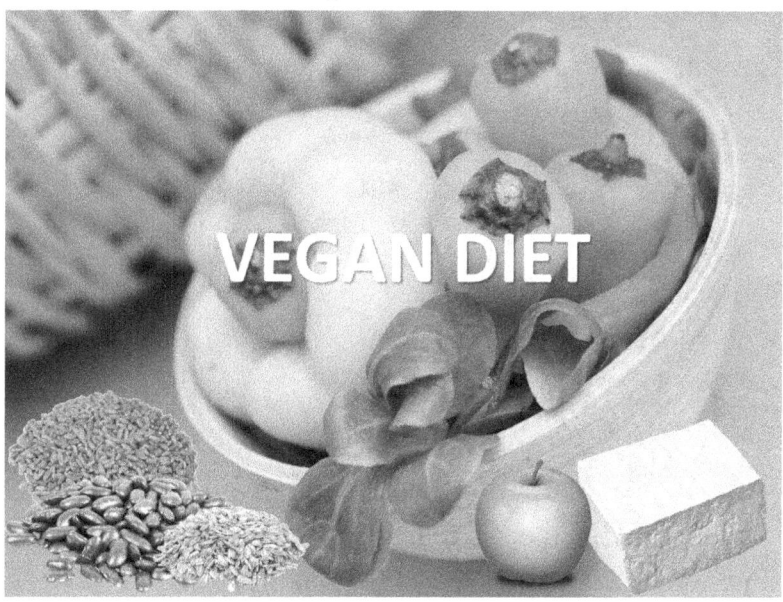

A vegan is a strict vegetarian. They don't eat any animal products at all. No eggs, no cheese or milk from cows. It also means that you have to pay close attention to the labels on some products. You might be surprised what food products contain animal-based elements.

For example, gelatin is made from the bones of animals. Gelatin is in marshmallows, which you might otherwise believe are purely sugar. A pure vegan won't eat honey because it comes from bees. A vegan is the most challenging of the plant-based diet approaches. However, as you'll see, there is still an abundance of options.

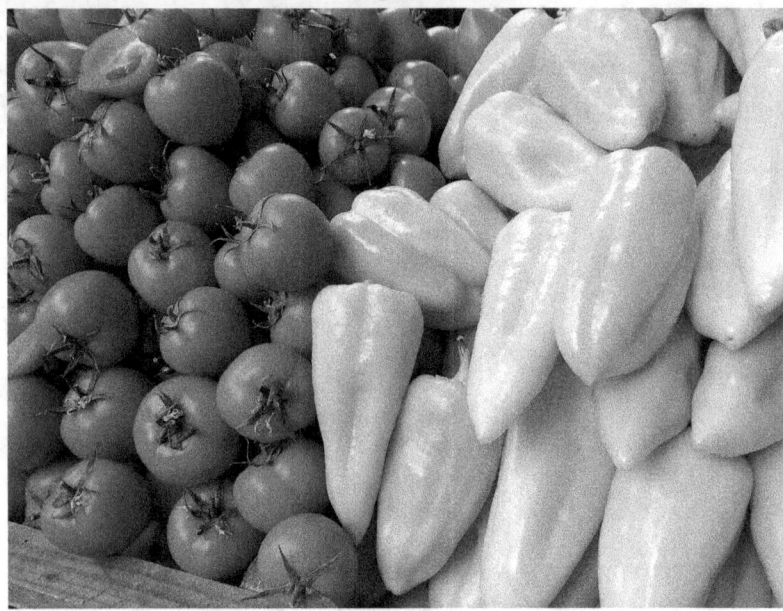

People who call themselves "vegans" will not eat any animal meat or anything derived from animals, such as milk and eggs. This means that they do not eat red meat, white meat, fowl, or any type of fish. Dairy products and eggs are off limits as well. They do not consume any kind of gelatin, honey or beeswax for food and don't use products derived from animals, such as leather, wool, or silk. Animal byproducts of any kind are avoided by vegans whose diet consists of fruits, vegetables, beans, and legumes. They try to eat foods as fresh as possible from the source of where they were grown or produced.

- Vegans do not consume any animal products, including, red meat, white meat (pork), fish, seafood, and poultry.

- They also exclude any foods derived from or made with animal products or byproducts, such as milk, yogurt, cheese, mayonnaise, butter, honey, gelatin, and eggs.

- Vegans also do not use any non-food products made from animals, such as beeswax, cosmetics, supplements, silk, leather, or wool.

Like any vegetarian diet, it is hoped that the convert will receive benefits such as weight loss, and the reduction of the risk of diabetes and heart disease, but for vegans it is more about following a philosophy rather than a diet.

According to the American Vegan Association, "veganism is compassion in action." It goes beyond a diet; it is a lifestyle and a philosophy. Veganism follows a "Reverence for Life" that recognizes the rights of all living creatures and nonviolence towards animals and the Earth.

They eat solely from the plant world and follow a generally healthy lifestyle and harmonious living. Animal rights groups are strong advocates of this type of philosophy, and many follow a vegan diet.

The vegan diet includes all plant foods, such as grains, fruit, nuts, and legumes. Soy products such as tofu, soymilk, and veggie burgers are commonly eaten. Soy can be a staple of the diet because it is a complete protein unlike other vegetable protein foods.

Other substitutes for meat products include almond milk, coconut milk, oat milk, and rice milk. Cheese substitutes include nutritional yeast, as well as products made from soy and tapioca. There are even egg substitutes such as silken tofu.

Lacto Vegetarian Diet

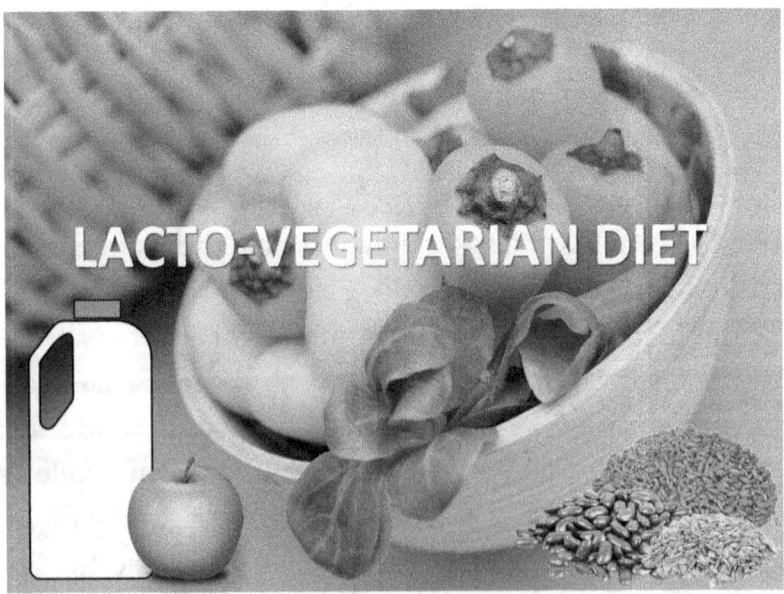

These people choose not to eat red meat, white meat, fowl, fish, or eggs. They get their protein from beans, legumes and dairy products of various types such as milk, cheese, yogurt, and other dairy products that come from cows or other grazing animals.

The lacto vegetarian diet excludes meat of all kind, but does allow dairy, like milk and cheese. This type of diet is popular among religious groups such as Hindus and Buddhists, and many Westerners.

The lacto vegetarian does not consume eggs because it contains future life and meat is avoided since its consumption would involve the taking of a life.

The consumption of dairy products helps the lacto vegetarian to meet his/her calcium requirements, which can be more difficult in the vegan diet. Dairy products, such as milk, yogurt, and cheese, are common milk products included in the lacto-vegetarian diet.

Ovo Vegetarian Diet

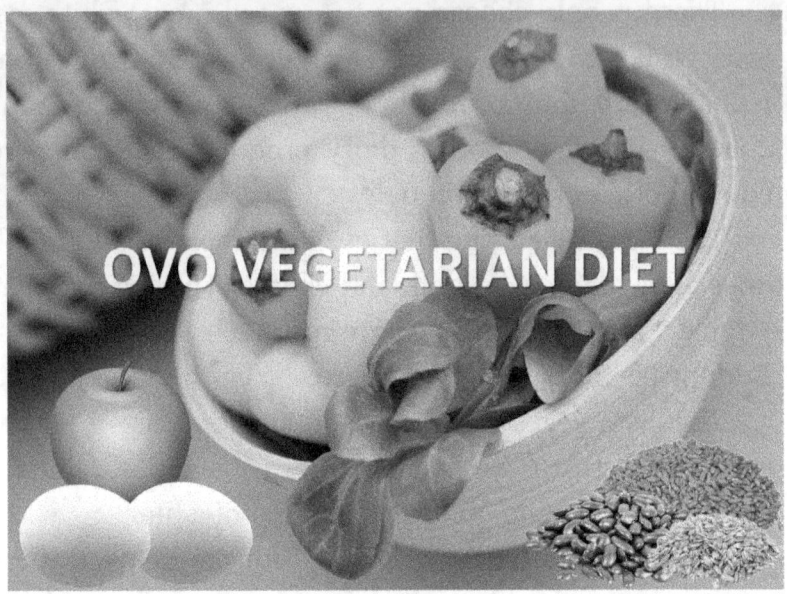

People who avoid eating red meat, white meat, fowl, and fish, but not eggs are known as ovo vegetarians. They also choose not to drink or eat dairy products derived from meat sources. For extra protein, ovo vegetarians eat fresh eggs from various types of fowl. Eggs are perfect sources of protein to aid the ovo vegetarian in the quest for a diet that provides enough protein to sustain them.

Ovo-vegetarians do not eat red or white meat, fish, poultry, seafood or dairy, but they do include eggs in their diet.

Lacto-ovo Vegetarian Diet

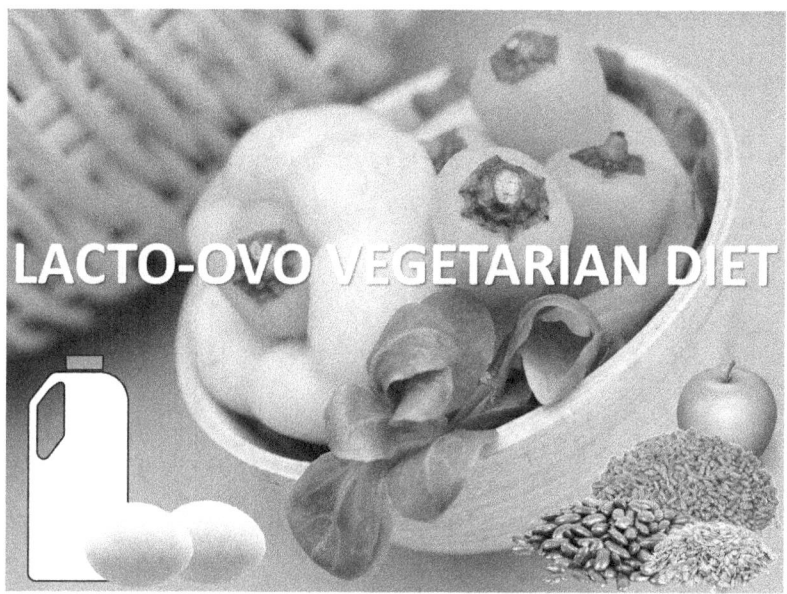

This is a vegetarian who elects not to eat red meat, white meat, poultry, or fish. They do, however, eat eggs and dairy products such as milk, cheese, and yogurt that come from cows and other grazing animals. This provides them with a wider base to choose from when getting protein into their system. Besides eggs and dairy products, beans and legumes can be excellent sources of dietary protein. It should be noted that most vegetarians are this type of vegetarian.

Like the lacto vegetarian, the lacto-ovo vegetarian has the advantage over more strict vegetarians of accessibility to calcium and zinc. This plan is popular among religious groups who eschew meat. Many seventh-day Adventists are followers of this diet.

If your diet is heavy in these elements right now, or if you're an athlete who needs a good deal of protein in your daily diet, then this approach may be the right choice for you. You can have whey protein drinks, eat eggs for breakfast, and have the occasional piece of cheese.

Pescatarian Vegetarian

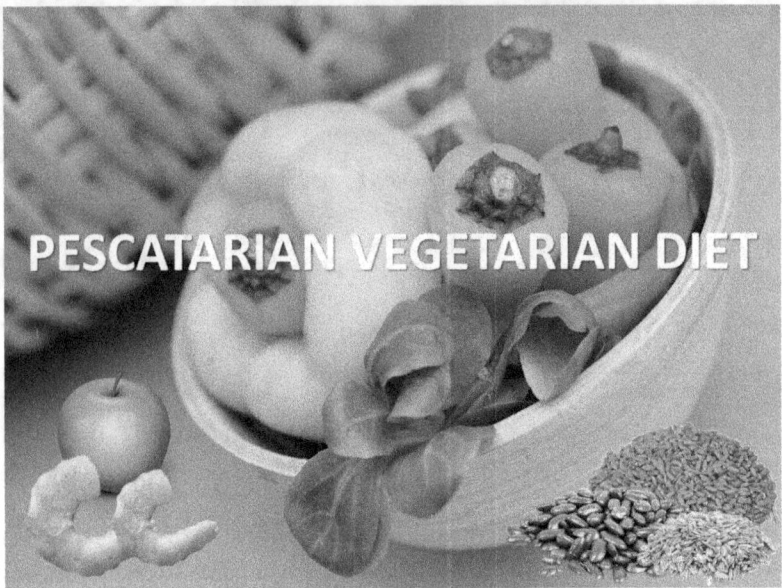

You might be surprised just how many vegetarians eat seafood and fish. So they don't eat beef, pigs, chickens, or any other two or four-legged animal, but they do eat fish. If you love seafood or want to occasionally have an option to eat "meat" then this may be a good option for you.

This plan includes seafood and fish along with a diet high in fruits, grains, and vegetables. The seafood provides quality protein, along with essential fatty acids to help build the cell walls in the body. Pescatarian do not eat poultry, red meat, or white meat. Some eat dairy and some do not.

Pollotarian Vegetarian

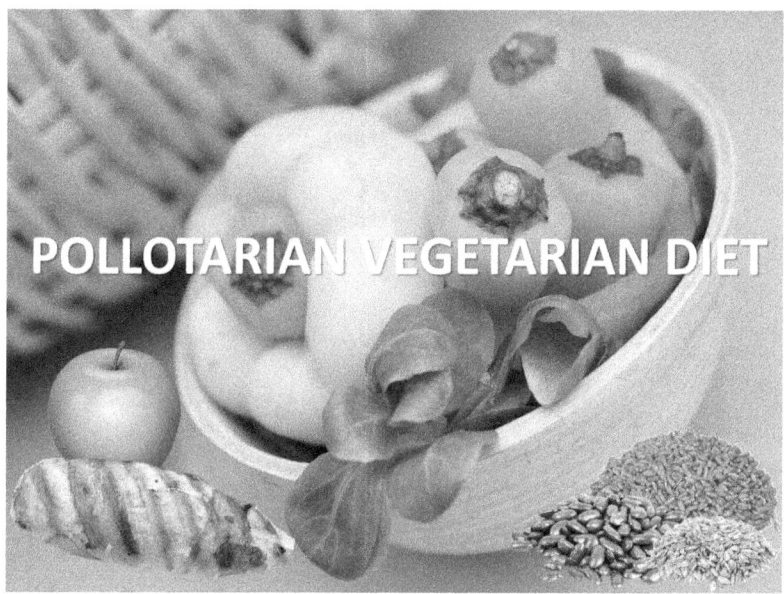

This is another partly vegetarian diet in which the person eliminates any type of red meat from the diet, but does include turkey, chicken, and other poultry along with fruits, vegetables, beans, legumes, and other non-meat items. They may or may not eat fish, seafood, and dairy.

Flexitarian Vegetarian

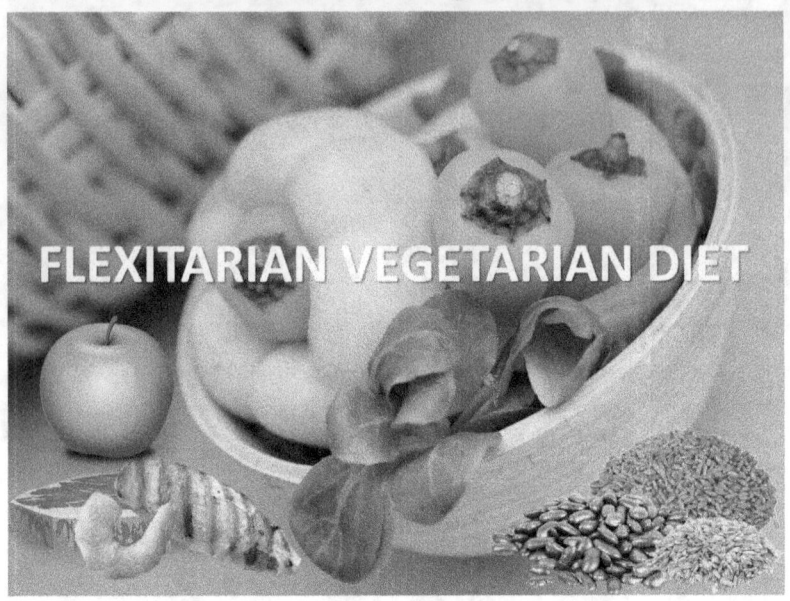

Here's where it can get a little more comfortable for many people. A flexitarian is someone who occasionally eats meat. So maybe you're a vegetarian 29 days of the month, but one day each month you eat meat. Or maybe you eat meat on Saturdays and you're a vegetarian the rest of the time. Again, the choice you make depends very much on what your goals and motivations are.

Finally, let's say that some vegetarians eat fish, eggs and dairy. They're still vegetarians. And let's also admit that as you begin this path toward a different way of eating, your approach may be different than how others approach it. You may decide to go all in and completely eliminate all animal-based products.

Or you might decide that that Friday night fish fry isn't something that you want to give up, so you eat meat once a week. Think about how you tend to set goals that you're successful at. Are you the type to go cold turkey or do you like to ease into transitions? Think about your current lifestyle. Does it support you to go cold turkey or should you adapt gradually?

Finally, it's okay to slip up. Forgive yourself and move forward. On that note, let's take a look at your new food groups. Meat is gone and there's a whole huge world of foods just waiting for your attention.

The flexitarian gets most of their nutrition from plant-based sources like fruits, vegetables, nuts, beans, and legumes. They will occasionally include various meat products as part of their diet but do not do so on a regular basis.

Plant-Based Diet Glossary

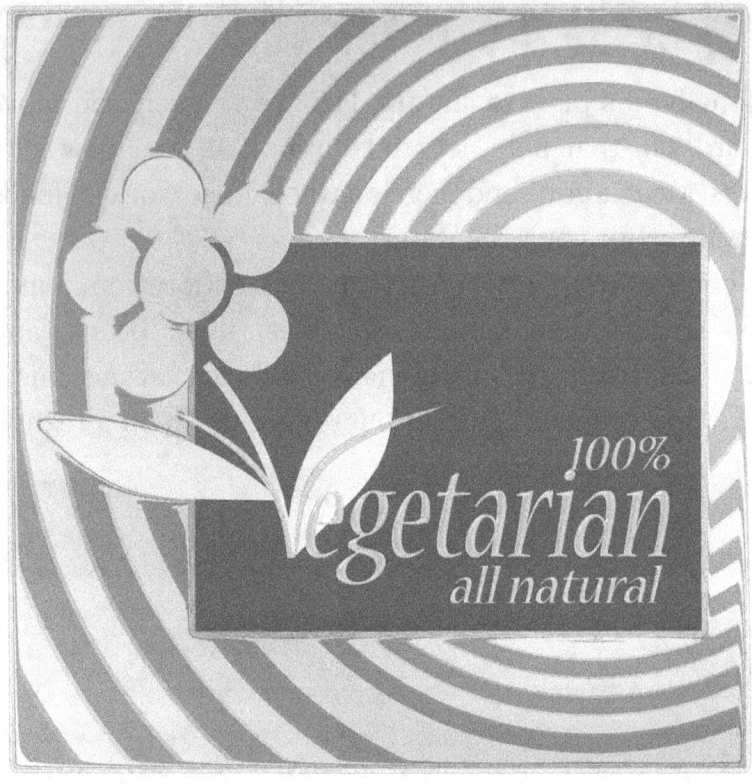

There is a special language for just about any sizable market or field. Heart doctors use different terminology than motorcycle enthusiasts. The same can be said for vegetarians, vegans and others that enjoy a plant-based diet. Refer to this handy glossary the next time you run up against a plant-based word or phrase that has you stumped. (Where applicable, a definition or process has been explained in depth to increase your level of knowledge.)

B12* (Cobalamin) - A coenzyme that is part of the metabolic process of every cell in the human body. This vitamin is essential for proper health. B12 is one of the 13 vitamins found naturally occurring in human beings. It is of the 8 B vitamins, and one of the most lacking of all nutrients in a plant-based diet. Trace amounts are found in mushrooms, seaweed and other plants, but a daily supplement is the only way to guarantee you are taking in healthy levels of this vital nutrient. Nutritional yeast is also a viable source of vitamin B12.

Calcium* - This mineral is crucial for building and maintaining strong, healthy bones. Calcium can be found in many plant-based foods. However, they do not exist in large enough quantities to fulfill most calcium recommendations. Food sources found in a plant-based approach to nutrition include mustard greens, broccoli, tempeh, beans and almonds.

D* - Vitamin D is a fat soluble secosteroid which aids in the healthy absorption of calcium, magnesium, zinc, iron and phosphate in humans. Like calcium, it is linked to bone health. Since the only source of this vital building block of health is through the action of sunlight hitting your skin, you are urged to supplement, or make sure you are getting 15 to 30 minutes of sunlight exposure on your skin every day.

Flaxseed - These seeds are either brown or yellow/gold in color (also known as golden linseeds). Flaxseeds are high in protein, dietary fiber, B vitamins, magnesium and phosphorous. They also contain Omega 3 fatty acids, and have been used as traditional Austrian medicines for treating gout, flu, rheumatism and infections. They are extremely versatile, and pound for pound an excellent source of nutrition and health.

Flexitarian - This word was created by combining the words flexible and vegetarian. This person can be regarded as a "semi-vegetarian", a plant-based eater most of the time, while occasionally eating meat.

Iron* - Iron is the most common element found on earth. Unfortunately, it does not make its way into plant eaters' bodies in sufficient quantity in most cases. Since it helps your body create red blood cells, it is extremely important to your health. Get enough iron in your diet and your skin and hair are strong and healthy. Your blood also effectively carries oxygen throughout your body. White beans, kidney beans, chickpeas, lentils and spinach are iron-rich.

Nutritional yeast - Often found in flake or powdered form, nutritional yeast is grown from sugar cane and molasses. It is a deactivated yeast that is often used to replace cheese, and is rich in B vitamins. It is gluten-free, has zero sodium, and makes a healthy gravy replacement for plant-based eaters. Beware of nutritional yeast (called "nooch" by vegans) that contains whey.

Omega 3 fatty acids* - Not all fats are bad. Your body requires healthy fatty acids. Omega 3s are unfortunately lacking from most diets, whether plant or meat-based. These fatty acids prevent heart disease and strokes, fight depression and anxiety, regulate a healthy blood pressure and are vital to a healthy nervous system. Crushed flax seeds and walnuts are two of the few plant-based sources of Omega 3s. A daily or weekly supplement is highly recommended.

Pescetarian - If you eat no meat, but eat fish, you are a pescetarian. Some vegetarians recognize the incredible health properties that fish like salmon deliver, so they supplement a veggie-based diet with fish. This provides healthy Omega 3 fatty acids that are often lacking in a vegetarian diet.

Seitan - This plant-based beef and meat replacement is made from cooked wheat gluten. It is high in protein and known in vegetarian and vegan circles as "wheat meat". The texture and look approximates beef and other meats when cooked, and it is a versatile part of many plant-centered diets.

Soy - Soy is both maligned and revered, depending on who you talk to. There are fermented and unfermented varieties. This vegetarian animal protein replacement is taken from soybeans. When you purchase soy, make sure it has been fermented, and is not the processed, unfermented version found in many soy-based milks, cheeses, burgers and ice creams linked to cancers and reproductive issues. A sensitivity to soy is one of the most common food allergies.

TVP - TVP stands for Textured Vegetable Protein. It is a refined, processed meat alternative that causes digestive problems in some. It is also called textured soy protein, and is created when soybean oil is extracted. This high-protein plant-based food is often considered less than healthy, so do your research before you add it to your diet.

Tempeh - This meat replacement hails from Indonesia. It is a staple in Asia and has been for hundreds of years. Tempeh is a fermented soybean-based food, extremely high in protein and calcium. Unlike tofu, it has a flavor and texture all its own. If you dislike the bland taste of tofu, tempeh may be worth a try.

Tofu (Bean Curd) - Tofu is almost synonymous with vegetarianism. It is made from soy milk, and is usually found in block form. There are soft, firm and extra-firm varieties. It is perfect for savory or sweet dishes because it has a tendency to absorb the flavors of the foods it is cooked with. Traced back to the Han dynasty in China over 2,000 years ago, tofu is still used extensively in Asia. It is a high-protein meat, egg and cheese alternative for a plant-centric diet.

Vegan - Veganism is "both the practice of abstaining from the use of animal products, particularly in diet, and an associated philosophy that rejects the commodity status of animals." Vegans will not eat, wear, purchase or knowingly possess any animal-based product. The term was coined in 1944 by Donald Watson, co-founder of The Vegan Society in England. A vegan is a vegetarian, but most vegetarians are not vegans.

Vegetarian - A vegetarian eats no meat, even fish. All vegetarians focus their nutrition on a plant-based approach. Some adopt this lifestyle for health, others for ethical or religious reasons. Variations include pescetarians (eats fish but no other meat), octo-vegetarians (eats eggs but no dairy products), lacto-vegetarians (eats dairy but no eggs) and octo-lacto-vegetarians (eats dairy and eggs), all of whom eat predominantly plants.

Zinc* - This mineral is important for the proper functioning of your immune and nervous systems. It also helps maintain healthy skin. A zinc deficiency is rather widespread, among plant-based eaters and those who consume a modern-day diet of processed and fast foods. Swiss chard, beans, pumpkin and sesame seeds and tofu are good sources of plant-based zinc.

When you restrict all animal meats from your diet, you could be missing out on important nutrients. Accordingly, nutritionists and health professionals alike agree there are several nutrients lacking from most plant-based diets. We have marked those above with an "*", so be sure to monitor your personal levels and supplement accordingly.

Reasons People Stop Eating

Meat

There are many reasons that a person might stop eating meat and meat products. They range from environmental too ethical to health reasons.

Health Benefits

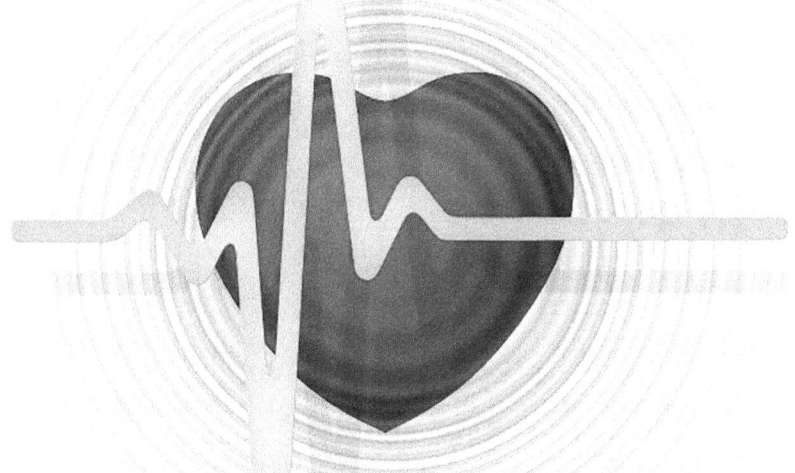

People are increasingly conscious of the benefits of health and exercise, especially with the countless research data that shows lifestyle choices to be key in preventing serious diseases such as cardiovascular disease, and type 2 diabetes. Studies show that vegetarian diets provide several important health benefits and can prevent chronic disease.

- **Prevent chronic disease** - People who eat a plant-based diet generally have lower cholesterol and blood pressure levels. They typically have lower risks for heart disease, type 2 diabetes, stroke, and cancers, while those who consume meat on a regular basis are at a higher risk.

- **Lower risk for heart disease** - One study (Tim Key, Director of The Cancer Epidemiology Unit at the University of Oxford, et al) looked at 45,000 volunteers (34% of whom were vegetarians) and showed "clear findings" that vegetarians have a 1/3 lower risk for heart disease than non-vegetarians.

- **Live longer** - The National Institutes of Health funded a study that allowed Loma Linda University, Loma Linda, California to continue ongoing research conducted into Seventh-day Adventists, named the Adventist Health Study 2. The study included 96,000 people from Canada and the United States and found that vegetarian men live an average of 9.5 years longer and vegetarian women and average of 6.1 years longer than meat eaters do. Pesco-vegetarians and semi-vegetarians who eat meat only once or week or so were found to have intermediate protection against lifestyle diseases.

Dr. Michael F. Roizen who wrote the book "Real Age Diet: Make Yourself Younger with What You Eat" says that you can add about 13 healthy years to your life with a plant based diet because animal foods clog heart arteries, destroy energy levels, and impact the health of the immune system.

A 30-year study that looked at residents of Okinawa, Japan, who have the longest life expectancy of any Japanese and really anyone from anywhere else in the world revealed the main stays of their diet to be comprised of fruits, vegetables, complex carbohydrates, and soy.

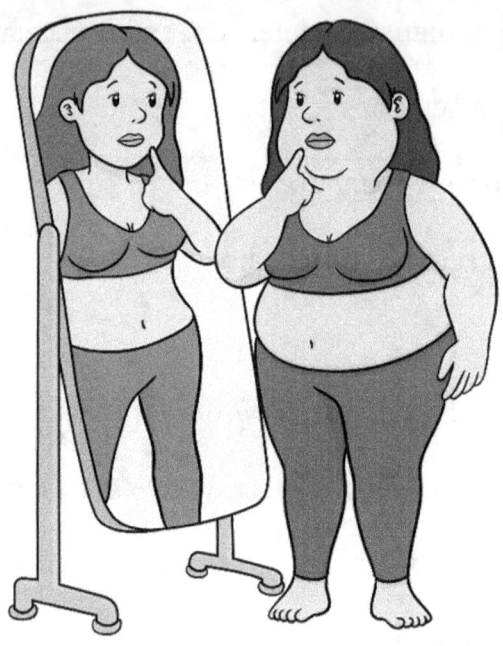

- **Weight management** - The Adventist Health Study 2 also showed that people who eat meat have a higher body weight for their age while vegans typically have the lowest, and on average, they are 30 pounds lighter. Vegans are also five units lighter on the BMI scale than those who eat meat.

- **Less insulin resistance** – According to the findings of the Adventist Health Study 2, both vegetarians and vegans are less insulin resistant than meat-eaters, thereby having a much lower risk for developing type 2 diabetes.

- **Avoid allergies** - Vegetarians are less likely to develop food allergies.

- **Avoid ingesting growth hormones** – Vegetarians who never eat meat, fish or poultry and vegans, never consume the growth hormones and antibiotics that are administered to farm animals raised for food production and passed on in food products to humans. The jury is still out as to the definitive effects of ingesting hormones and antibiotics, but many believe that at the very best, they are unnecessary for humans, and at the worst they cause harm that is yet to be discovered.

- **Better mood and increased energy** - High intake of plant foods results in a better mood, huge boost in energy, and feelings of calm and happiness.

- **Prevent cancer**- Plant foods contain essential antioxidants that prevent cell damage that can destroy cells or lead to mutations that cause various cancers.

- **Ease menopausal symptoms** – Plant foods are rich in phytoestrogens, which are chemical compounds that mimic the behavior of estrogen. A healthy balance of estrogen and progesterone levels in the diet facilities a more comfortable passage through menopause. Soy, a staple of the vegan diet is especially high in phytoestrogens, along with other plant foods like cherries, olives, berries, and apples. Additionally, vegetarian diets promote healthy weight management with a low fat, high fiber diet that can help prevent the typical weight gain seen in menopausal women.

- **Boost libido** - Plant foods contain libido-boosting properties, and vegetarian diets result in lower body weight that increases the release of sex hormones.

- **Vegetarian diets reduce the risk of contracting food-borne illnesses** - The Centers for Disease Control reports that there are 76 cases of food-borne illnesses each year in the United States that results in 325,000 hospitalizations and 5,000 deaths. The US Food and Drug Administration (FDA) reports that the main sources of food-borne illness are meat, poultry, fish, and seafood.

- **Avoid toxic chemicals** - The EPA estimates that nearly 95% of the pesticide residue in a typical American diet stems from meat, dairy and fish. Fish, in particular, contain carcinogens and heavy metals that cannot be eliminated through cooking or even freezing. Sometimes meat and dairy foods may be laced with hormones and steroids, making it that much more important to read food labels.

- **Boost digestive health** – Eating a high fiber plant diet improves and supports digestive health, and helps to prevent hemorrhoids, constipation, and diverticulitis.

Religion

Some religions are known for their avoidance of meat, these include but are not limited to, Hinduism, Jainism, Buddhism, and Seventh Day Adventists.

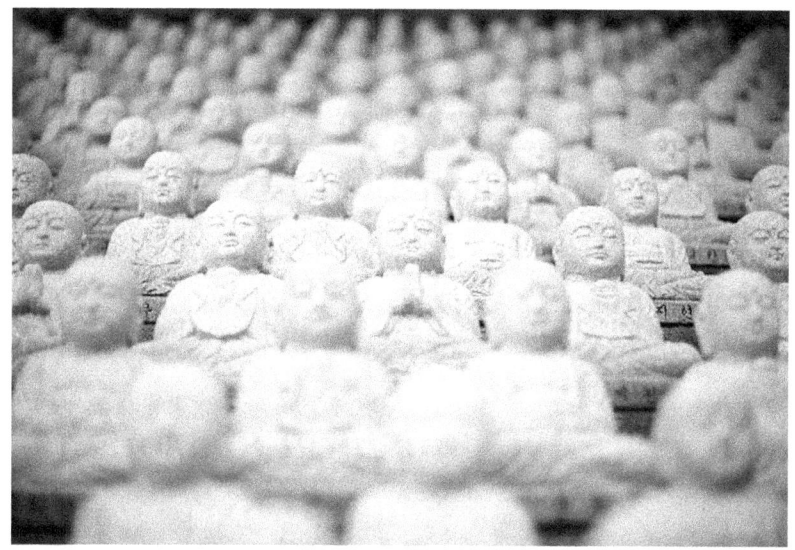

- Hindus believe that by avoiding meat, they are fulfilling their religious obligations. They also avoid meat for the reason of Karmic consequences.

- The central belief in Jainism is the avoidance of killing or harming any living creature.

- Some Buddhists don't eat meat, while others do, depending on their interpretation of Buddhist laws.

- Seventh-day Adventists are either lacto-ovo vegetarians, who avoid meat, but eat eggs and dairy or vegans. The philosophy behind this religion's recommendation to avoid meat is clearly stated, as "we believe God calls us to care for our bodies, treating them with the respect a divine creation deserves. Gluttony and excess, even of something good, can be detrimental to our health."

Environmental Reasons

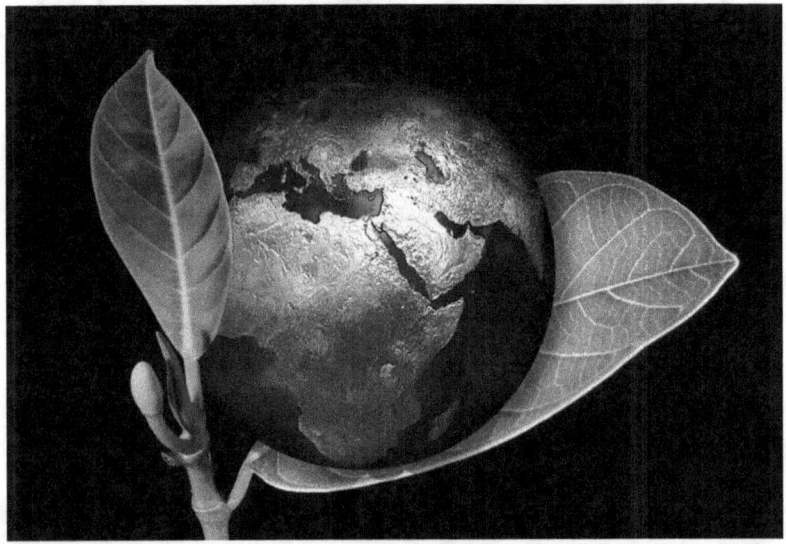

The world is abuzz with environmental concerns and eco-friendly lifestyles; appropriately, there are environmental reasons why people stop eating meat.

- Large areas of land are needed to raise animals, particularly cattle. It is believed that this land could be better put to use with the production of crops for consumption. Crops, like other plants, also prevent erosion from taking place on the Earth's land.

- Commercial animal waste that is not properly handled tends to end up in our rivers, eventually contaminating ground water supplies.

- Overgrazing may negatively affect wildlife species. Areas that were inhabited by wildlife are sacrificed for the use of raising animals for food, particularly cattle. Natural predators who are all part of the animal kingdom and contribute to a healthy eco-system are eliminated to protect domestic cattle from predation.

- The emission of greenhouse gases by livestock is another reason that some choose a vegetarian diet. It has been estimated that livestock emit 14.5% of the world's greenhouse gases.

Ethical Reasons

Ethical reasons that drive people to stop eating meat and meat products have grown recently as farming has become more advanced in developed countries and some of the horrors of farm animal slayings for human consumption have been highlighted in the media and by animal activist groups.

Many simply refuse to eat anything that had a mom.

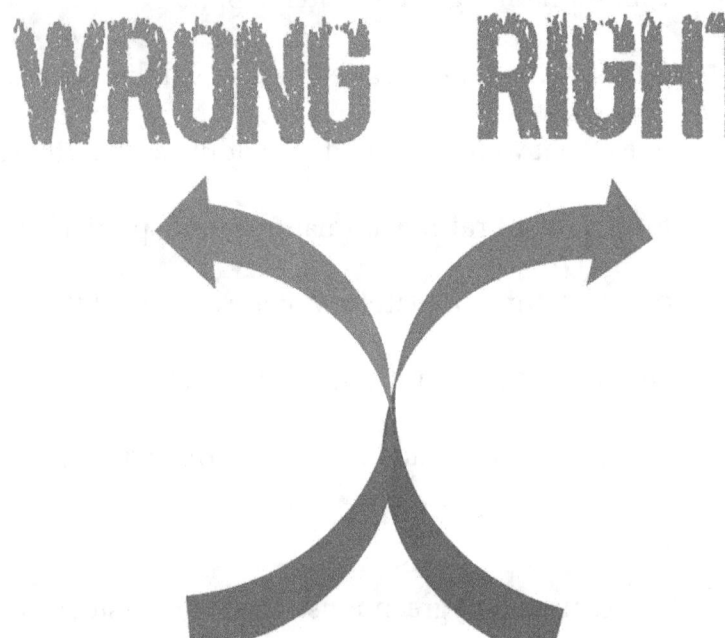

The ethical reasons include:

- The belief that killing an animal is like killing a human is one of the biggest ethical reasons

- The belief that animals feel the same emotions as humans and their non-humane slaughter for human food is not moral
- The belief that animals feel pain in the same way that humans do
- Some maintain that even the production of eggs and milk causes some suffering for young animals
- Premature death can and does occur, such as the case when calves are killed for the production of veal

The consumption of animals poses two moral problems that are endlessly debated in modern society:

- Is it morally wrong to raise animals with only the purpose of human consumption?
- Does it stop being wrong if the process is carried out in a human fashion?

For the vegan, the above answers are a firm yes and no respectively.

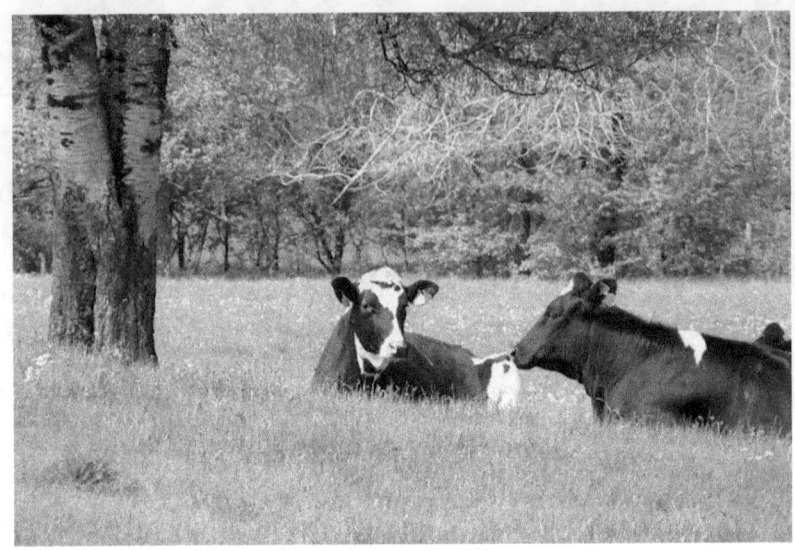

The Animal Rights Viewpoint

The basic premise to the humanitarian aspect of vegetarian living is that animals have rights, and so the raising and killing of animals for food is morally wrong. The hallmark of the moral issue is that when an animal is raised solely for the purpose of feeding humans, even when it is done so in a humane fashion, that animal is being treated as a means to human ends and not as an end in itself, which violates the animal's rights.

The rights of the animal refer to its interests, and the raising and slaughter of animals for food violates the animal's right to continue living.

This philosophy also maintains that modern farming and cattle raising methods violate key interests of all animals, including:

- Their rights to live in a natural and decent environment
- Their ability to make free choices
- To avoid pain and fear
- To graze in a natural environment and consume a natural diet
- To participate within the bounds of their natural habitat, which includes the social and community aspects of its species

The Hypocrisy Dilemma

In its simplest form, the ethical objection to eating animals stems from the viewpoint of a simple hypocrisy. We nurture, love and care for certain animals, like cats, dogs and even hamsters, while at the same time raise, and slaughter cows, pigs, calves and chickens for human consumption.

Those who challenge this hypocrisy raise a legitimate question: If we don't slaughter dogs and cats for food, then why is it okay to slaughter and eat other animals?

Food for thought.

Avoiding Growth Hormones from Meat

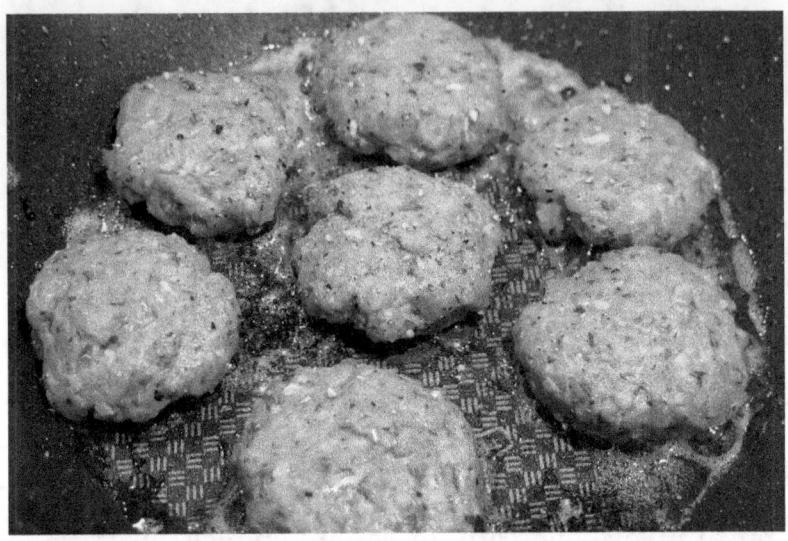

Another reason people choose to eat a plant diet is to avoid eating growth hormones from meat. Commercially raised cattle are given antibiotics and growth hormones, which the consumer ingests by eating these products. This is just another motivation behind eating a plant diet that eliminates meat.

Save Money

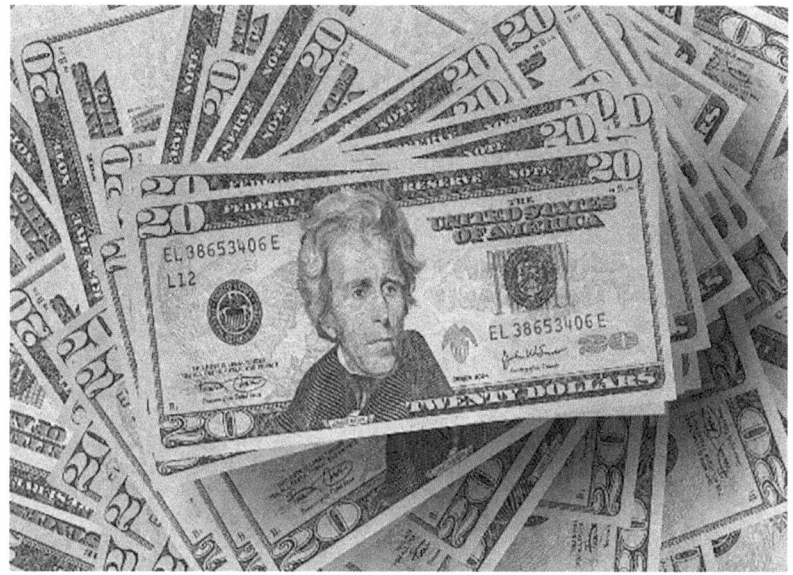

Did you know that meat accounts for 10% of American's food budgets? Replacing the nearly 200 pounds of meat non-vegetarians consume yearly with vegetables, grains, and fruits can cut the average food bill by an about $4,000 a year.

Humans Are by Nature Vegetarians

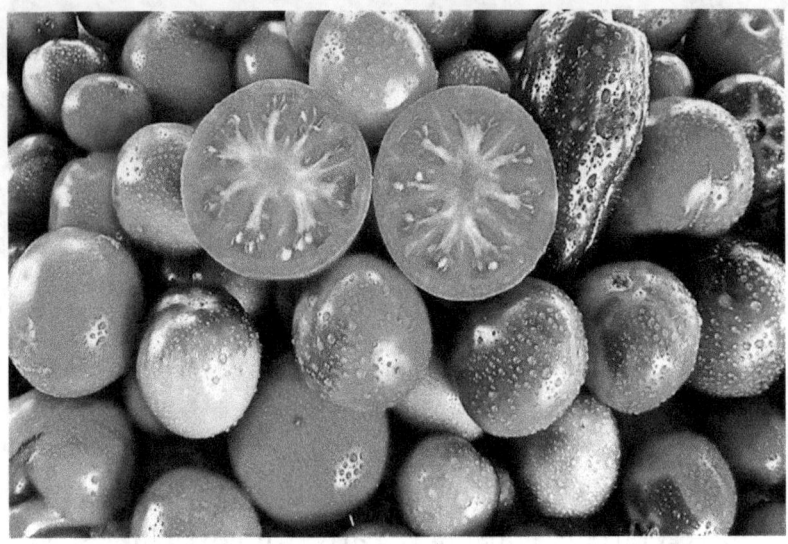

It is argued and believed by some that humans are vegetarians by nature because of the anatomical differences between carnivorous animals and humans. The proponents of this argument say that we have more in common with herbivores in areas like facial muscles, jaw type, teeth, saliva, and how we eat.

Health Benefits of Vegan and

Vegetarian Diets

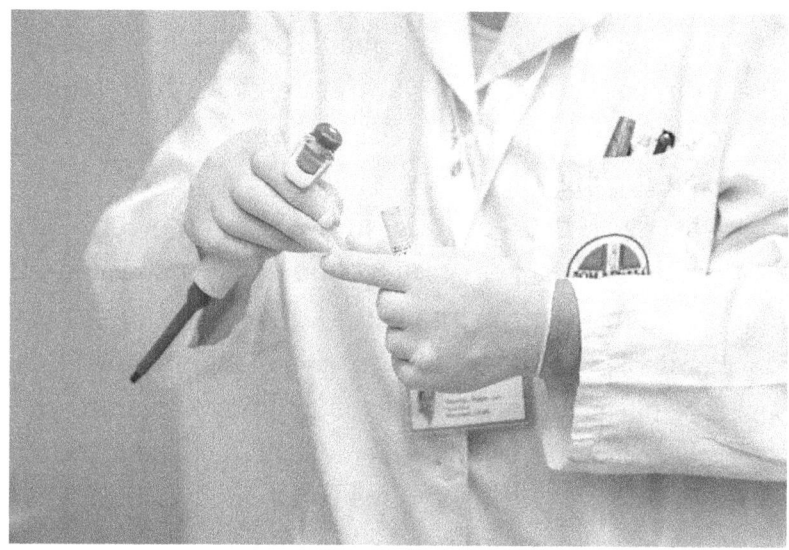

With all the advances in science and the loads of research that support lifestyle choice as the most successful method to prevent disease and possible premature death from such, many are taking heartfelt steps to make healthy choices in their diet, and exercise habits.

One of these studies done by the Harvard Medical School showed that male subjects who ate red meat five or more times a week had four times the risk of colon cancer than men who consumed it less than once a month.

Evidence exists vegetarian diets can help to prevent various chronic diseases and live a longer life. This occurs for various reasons, but a lot is attributed to the extraordinary nutrient density of plant foods. Plant foods are created by nature and provide not only healthy sustenance for the human body, they are also nutrient dense and offer a variety of micronutrients, including vitamins, minerals, and antioxidants along with the essential macronutrients, carbohydrates, protein and healthy fats.

The attributes of a plant-based diet cannot be overemphasized enough. Natural nutrients that come from earth foods help to nutrify the body, provide ample energy for even the busiest of lives and help to prevent disease in part because they contain ample amounts of essential antioxidants that help protect the cells of the body from damage caused by free radicals.

Plant-based diets can play a significant role in preventing certain types of chronic illness, including cancer, heart disease and type 2 diabetes. Plant diets also help to prevent obesity and its serious consequences and facilitate weight loss, along with improving digestive health.

However, plant foods go beyond in that they exclude harmful elements the body does not need, and in this way help to support human health even further.

Some of the other ways that increasing your intake of plant food can help you include lower instances of heart disease, which is the leading killer of both men and women in the United States, stroke, neural tube defects, and diabetes.

Plant foods also carry less risk of foodborne illnesses, are better for the environment, and often offer more natural flavors than animal proteins do.

Protection Against Cancer

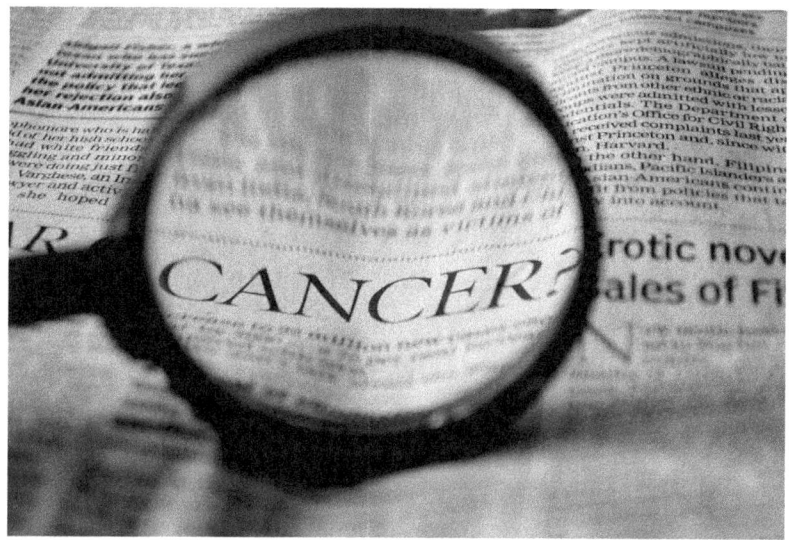

Cancer of various types affects millions of people across the world. There are mild forms of cancer such as basal cell cancer and squamous cell cancer of the skin, and more serious types of cancer, including lung cancer, colon cancer and breast cancer. Cancers have many different causes and increasingly, scientists and researchers are noticing that a person's dietary habits contribute to getting certain forms of cancer.

For example, both breast cancer and colon cancer are linked to diets containing high amounts of saturated fats from meat sources. They have found that vegetarians have lower rates of cancer from these sources when compared to meat-eaters. Those who are at an especially high risk for these cancers may have a therapeutic reason to adopt a vegetarian lifestyle, such as avoiding the saturated fats found in meat and chicken.

Recent studies have shown that colorectal cancer is linked to the consumption of processed red meat. It has been reported that the risks of this type of cancer increased by 20% to 29% depending on the amount of red meat ingested.

The process of cooking red meat can also increase the risk of cancer. Cooking red meat over an open fire, or at a high temperature has been shown to produce powerful carcinogens. Grilling, frying, and smoking are methods commonly used to cook meats that fall into this category.

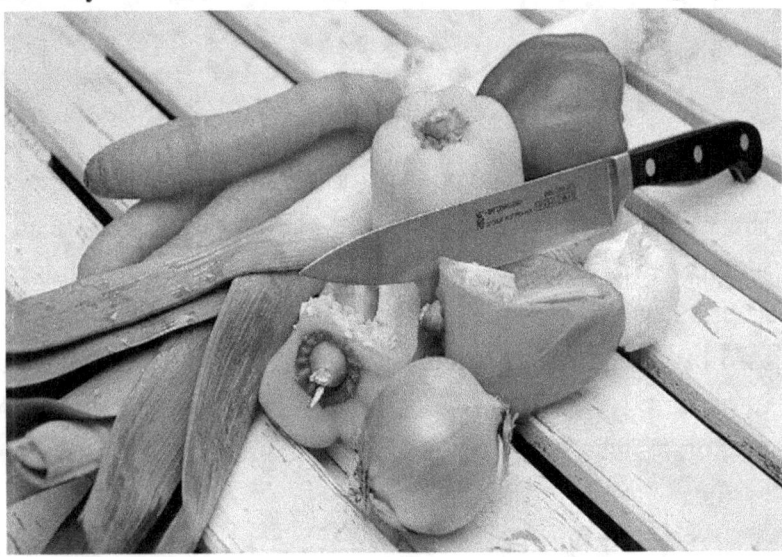

It has also been shown that a high protein intake associated with eating meat increased the risk of cancer compared to eating vegetable protein.

Both breast cancer and colon cancer are also linked to diets that include an excessive amount of saturated fats from meat sources. Statistics show that vegetarians have lower incidence rates of these cancers when compared to those who eat meat.

Obesity and Cancer

Vegetarians tend to consume fewer calories than non-vegetarians do and therefore are leaner than those people who eat meat. Obesity is linked to both breast cancer and colon cancer—something that can be avoided when a person adopts a vegetarian diet and maintains a healthy weight. It is believed that people who already have cancer may have a better chance for survival if they eat a vegetarian diet, although the data on this is somewhat scarce.

Obesity is linked to both breast cancer and colon cancer—something that can be avoided when a person adopts a vegetarian diet and maintains a healthy weight. It is believed that people who already have cancer may have a better chance for survival if they eat a vegetarian diet, although the data on this is somewhat scarce.

Plant Foods and Antioxidants

Vegetables and fruits are also high in antioxidants, which are molecules that neutralize oxygen free radicals in the body. Oxygen free radicals can damage all parts of a human cell, including the DNA from those cells. Damaged DNA translates to cellular death or a mutation in the cell that leads to cancer. Fruits such as blueberries and other berries are especially high in antioxidants and should be included as part of a therapeutic/preventative vegetarian diet.

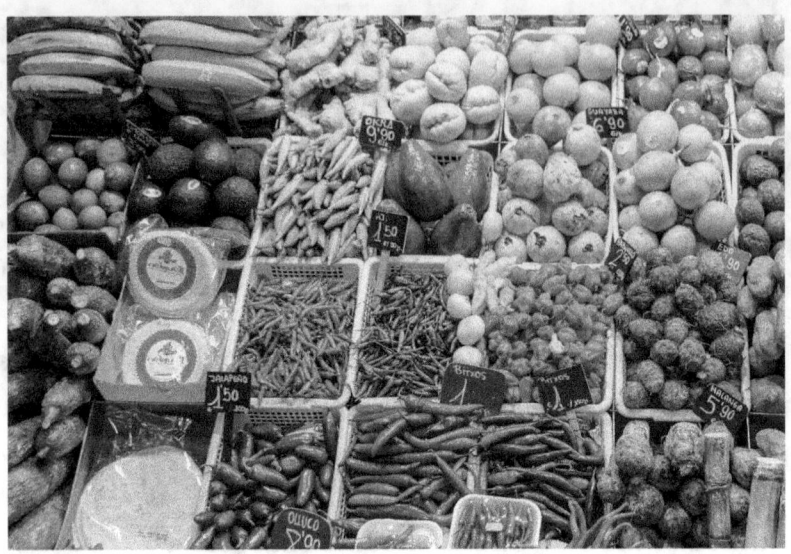

There had initially been concerns on the part of scientists and doctors about women eating soy products if they have or are at risk for breast cancer. This is because soy products contain a great amount of plant estrogens, which were thought to make cancer cells from the breasts grow and develop. Newer research on plant estrogens such as those derived from soybeans have shown no effect of eating these types of foods or a possible slight benefit from eating soy bean products while having breast cancer. This includes foods like tofu and soymilk, which can be mainstays of a vegetarian diet, providing good protein sources.

Other Plant Sources of Antioxidants

- Cranberries
- Nuts and especially walnuts, pistachios, pecans, hazelnuts and almonds

- Sunflower, sesame and flaxseeds
- Beans: kidney beans, black beans, pinto beans and lentils
- Edamame
- Prunes
- Purple, red and blue grapes
- Dark Green Vegetables: kale, spinach, artichokes, broccoli, okra and others
- Red Delicious, Granny Smith and Gala apples
- Pears
- Pecans
- Sweet cherries
- Chocolate (at least 60% cacao)
- Russet potatoes and sweet potatoes with skin on
- Plums
- All orange and red vegetables
- Green tea
- Whole grains

Adopting a Vegetarian Diet

There are many research articles showing the benefit of eating a vegetarian diet in the prevention of cancer. When you adopt a vegetarian diet, you get most of your nutrients from fruits and vegetables as well as soy products, whole grain foods, beans and legumes. No red meat, white meat, or poultry products are included in a vegetarian diet and many vegetarians choose not to eat fish. This is an eating strategy that will especially benefit those who, by virtue of heredity or other lifestyle factors, find themselves at a higher than average risk of getting cancer.

Before adopting a strict vegetarian diet, such as a vegan diet, speak to your doctor about getting a referral to see a nutritionist who will help you find food guides that fit with a vegetarian diet. Purchase a vegan or vegetarian cookbook to help guide you toward recipes that are healthy, high in nutrients and contain no meat products. The research on things like eggs and milk or dairy products is less strong than it is on eating animal meat itself so you can choose whether you want to include cheese, eggs, yogurt, and milk in your vegetarian diet.

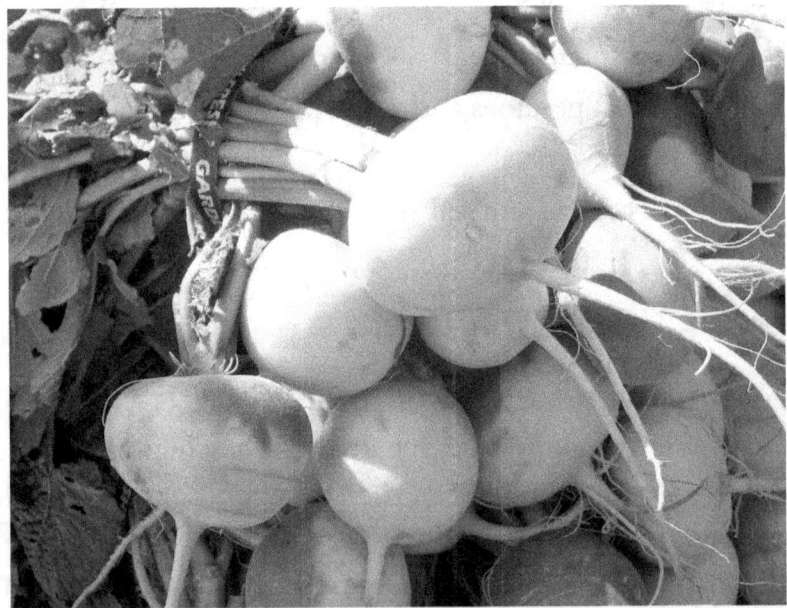

Glucosinolates

Cruciferous vegetables are part of a genus of plants that contain glucosinolates, which are known to have anti-cancer properties. Studies have shown that people who consume cruciferous vegetables regularly have lower risks of colorectal cancer, breast cancer and lung cancer.

Bok choy, Brussel sprouts, turnips, cabbage, kale, and cauliflower are just some of the plants that fall within this group.

Heart Disease

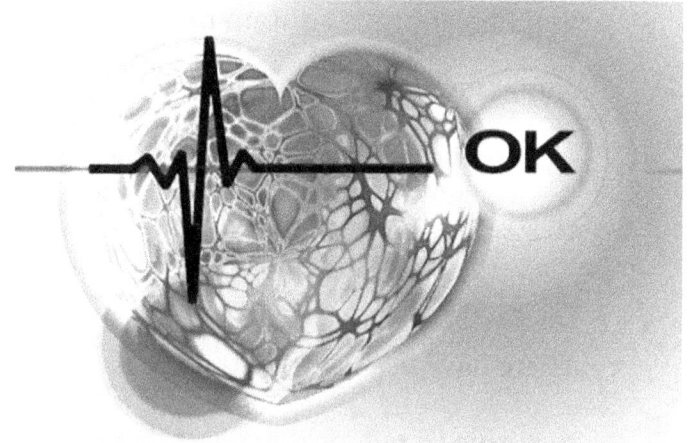

It turns out that vegetarians have advantages when it comes to getting heart disease, including heart attacks and strokes. Vegetarian diets are beneficial for heart disease for several reasons, including the following:

- **A vegetarian diet is low in saturated fat.** Most saturated fats in the diet come from meats and vegetarians, by definition, do not eat meat. They get some fat in dairy products if they choose to have dairy in their diet and plant oils contain unsaturated fats, which are much healthier for you. Saturated fat often turns into cholesterol, which lines the arteries in critical places, causing blockages of arteries supplying the heart, the brain and the peripheral vascular system. Vegetarian diets contain practically no cholesterol so arteries remain open and flowing to crucial body areas. Former meat eaters who choose to eat vegetarians can reduce arterial plaque.

- **There have been studies linking the substance L-carnitine in red meat to heart disease.** These studies show that this substance rather than the saturated fat and cholesterol in red meats is the culprit in increasing the risks. Bacteria that live in the stomach consume this substance and break it down into trimethylamine-N-oxide or TMAO, which leads to clogged arteries. Vegan and dairy free vegetarian diets are also naturally very low in cholesterol (unless the vegetarian over consumes baked goods, junk food or sweets), and this further supports heart health. The high fiber content helps to maintain low levels of the bad LDL cholesterol and increase the good HDL cholesterol.

- **Vegetarian diets are low in calories, thus combating obesity.** People who are obese carry a greater risk of heart disease. Adopting a no meat, vegetarian diet can promote weight loss and reduce the risk of obesity-related diseases. People who eat a vegetarian diet can reduce their body mass index to 25 or less. A normal weight person has a body mass index of between 18 and 25, as calculated by taking the weight in pounds and dividing it by the height in inches, and multiplying that number by 703. This is a calculated number worth knowing if you are at risk for heart disease by virtue of family history, hypertension, or other risk factors.

- **Vegetarian diets are high in soluble fiber.** Soluble fiber in the diet can absorb any cholesterol that might otherwise be absorbed into the system and contribute to arterial plaque. Great sources of soluble fiber in a therapeutic vegetarian diet are found in barley, whole grains, vegetables, beans, and apples. All of these foods are welcome in a vegetarian diet and will do double duty as good nutrition and in lowering cholesterol.

- **Plants consist of healthy oils.** Plants contain healthy oils that provide your body with necessary fatty acids without the saturated fat found in animal fats. Even a vegetarian diet needs a certain amount of fat in order to promote cell wall growth, for brain health and other vital chemical processes in the body.

Vegetarians who try to exclude unsaturated fat from their diet will not be as healthy as those who put plant oils in as part of the vegetarian program. Plant oils are fats taken from the seed of plants, they include: avocado seed oil, coconut oil, flax seed oil, grapeseed oil, hemp oil, olive oil,

Safflower seed oil, sesame seed oil, and soybean oil, just to name a few.

- **There are other plant chemicals healthy for the heart and which combat heart disease.** The risk of heart attack and stroke is further lessened by eating fruits and vegetables containing phytosterols and other plant antioxidants. There is much research left to be done on how plants exactly prevent heart disease but it is believed that the molecules and phytonutrients in a vegetarian diet help fight heart disease in many different ways.

- Plant foods for heart health.

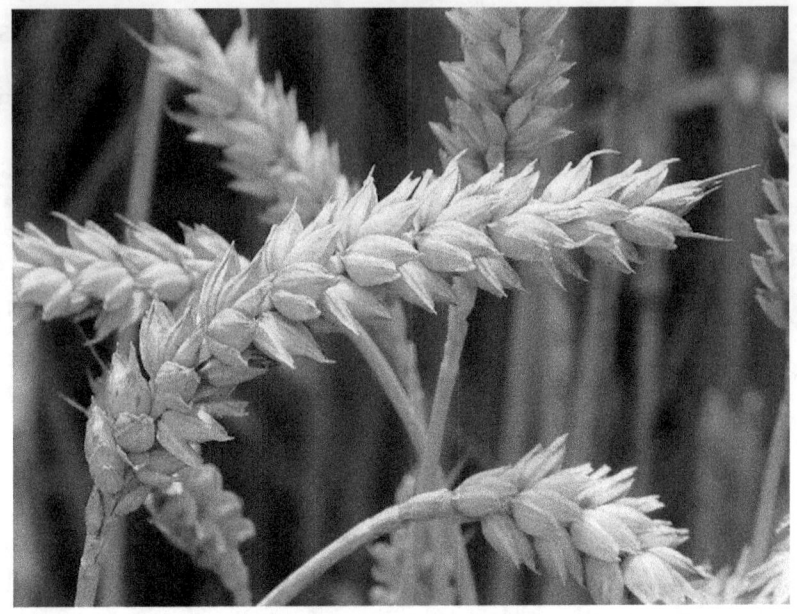

- Oats contain high levels of fiber, which lowers bad LDL cholesterol. This prevents the clogging of heart arteries that can lead to heart attack, premature death and the need for bypass surgery. Oats also contain potassium, which lowers blood pressure. Steel cut oats are best and instant oats should be avoided because of their high sugar content.

- Blueberries contain fiber and anti-oxidants, which are also good for heart health.

- Soy, which is also rich in fiber, is known to prevent cardiovascular disease by lowering triglycerides. It has a high level of polyunsaturated fats, which is known to lower cholesterol levels. Soymilk, tofu, and edamame are popular forms of vegan soy protein.

- Dark chocolate contains polyphenols. This compound is known to lower blood pressure. It also lowers inflammation as well as clotting.

- Citrus fruits contain flavonoids, which are known to lower risks of cardiovascular problems.

- Nuts contain polyunsaturated fats, fiber and omega-3 fatty acids, all of which support heart health.

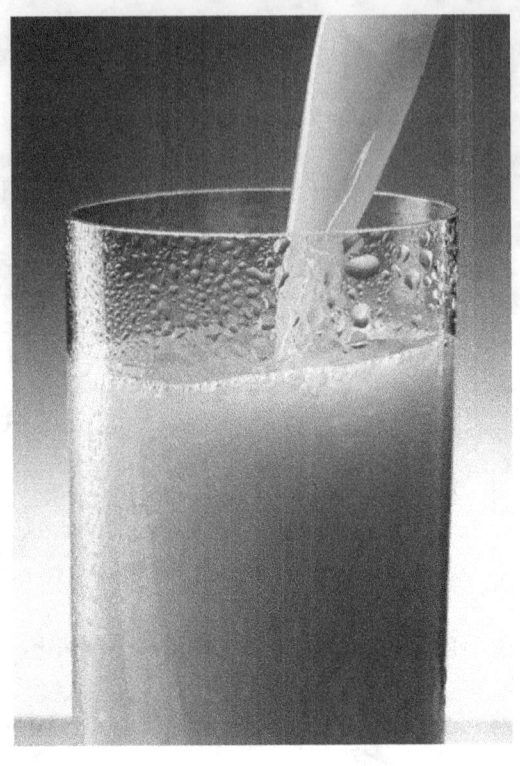

- Virgin olive oil is a heart healthy quality source of monounsaturated fats. A recent landmark study that analyzed people who follow the Mediterranean Diet, of which olive oil is a staple, showed a 30% reduction in deaths from heart disease for high risk patients. Healthy individuals enjoyed a 9% reduction rate for heart disease. It is also noteworthy to mention that the

Mediterranean diet limits red meat to once weekly.

- The risk of heart attacks and strokes is further lessened by a diet rich in fruits and vegetables that contain phytosterols and other plant antioxidants. Experts strongly believe that the actual molecules and phytonutrients in a vegetarian diet play a key role in fighting heart disease in many different ways.

Speak to your doctor or nutritionist about ways you can use a vegetarian diet as a way to reduce your heart disease risks.

Type 2 Diabetes

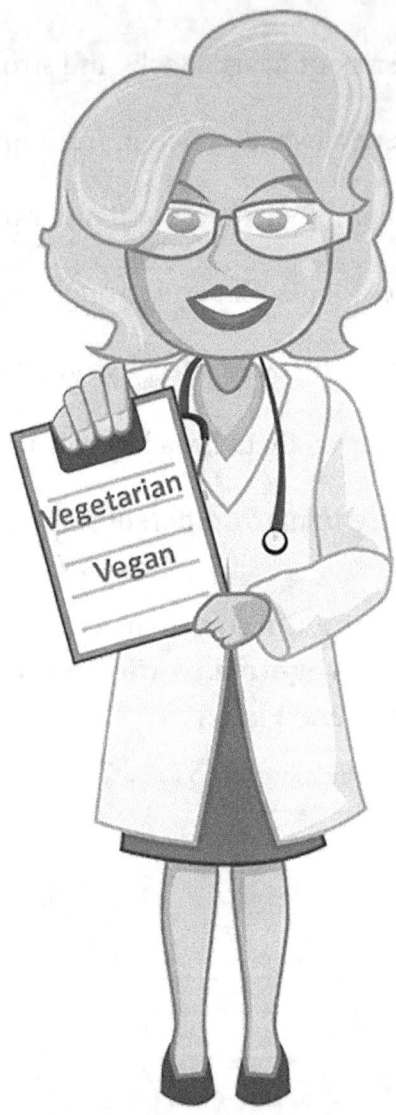

A vegetarian diet might be the best choice for people with type 2 diabetes. This is because vegetarian diets tend to be rich in complex carbohydrates, which have a low glycemic index. Foods with a low glycemic index, such as whole fruits and vegetables, usually contain fiber, which keeps simple sugars from flooding the bloodstream. On the other hand, diets with foods containing a high glycemic index often contain pastries, white bread, and sweets that will flood the bloodstream with sugar, overworking the pancreas, which is responsible for putting out insulin in response to the high sugar load. Studies show that vegetarians have improved insulin resistance and lower incidence of type 2 diabetes than those who are not.

Protein Needs for Those with Diabetes

Type 2 diabetics or those who are considered pre-diabetic need to have a non-meat source of valuable protein for a healthy, well-run body. Proteins make up almost all the enzymes needed by the body that run the various bodily functions. Fortunately, quality proteins exist in vegetarian diets that include plenty of legumes, beans, some vegetables, and sometimes dairy proteins. It all depends on what kind of vegetarian you are. If you are a lacto-ovo-vegetarian, it means that you eat eggs and milk created by farm animals. Both milk and eggs are high in protein, negating the need to eat the actual meat of a farm animal.

Weight Loss and Vegetarianism

Vegetarian diets are usually lower in calories than non-vegetarian diets. For type 2 diabetics, this can mean weight loss, which is geared toward improving the blood sugar numbers the diabetic gets when checking their hemoglobin A1C or their daily blood glucose values. A healthy vegetarian diet can easily contain between 1500 and 2000 calories, well within a range that will allow for a gradual weight loss of ten or more pounds over several weeks. Research has shown that weight loss as part of a vegetarian diet can decrease the amount of medication a type 2 diabetic must take in order to keep blood sugar numbers stable.

In fact, vegetarian diets that lead to weight loss can be all that mild type 2 diabetics need to keep the blood sugars within normal range and medications may be stopped or not started at all. The therapeutic advantage of a vegetarian diet has been shown in study after study on the topic of vegetarianism and type 2 diabetes.

How to Eat a Balanced Vegetarian Diet

For proper nutrition, vegetarian diabetics need all of these components in their diet:

- **Protein** from vegetarian sources such as beans and legumes or from dairy and eggs if that is your persuasion.

- **Carbohydrates** should be included mainly from vegetables. Additionally, fruits, and starches like whole grains should be consumed in moderation, while monitoring how your blood glucose levels react to such foods.

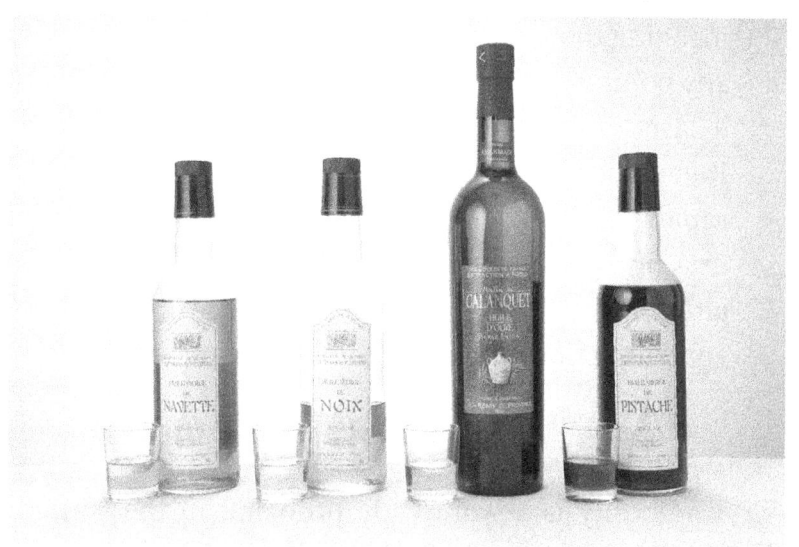

- **Healthy fats** (monosaturated, and polyunsaturated) need to be a part of every diet in small quantities. There are essential fatty acid supplements a diabetic can take that provide the necessary fat without the need for eating meat. Fat needn't be a large part of a diabetic vegetarian diet so a supplement can take care of all of the fatty acid needs.

Vegetarians who are also diabetic should consider eating several small meals per day, incorporating the three major macronutrients listed above. When you eat several small meals per day, the dose of complex carbohydrates is steady, meaning there are fewer spikes in blood sugar and insulin at any point in the day. The pancreas is never over-worked and it lasts longer without the added stress of glucose spikes. Remember that it's the glycemic index that controls the rapidity of glucose influx into the system. Look online for lists of foods and their glycemic index. You will find food alternatives to high sugar foods that will provide you with good nutrition without high blood sugar levels.

Obesity

Obesity is a worldwide problem, in the United States, alone the numbers have doubled since 2008 from 15% to 30% of the population. In the United States, obesity numbers are at an epidemic level. 68.5% of the US population is either overweight or obese with more than 2/3 of adults being overweight or obese in 2014. A normal weight is defined as having a body mass index (BMI) of 25 or less but greater than about 18. Fortunately, a vegetarian diet can address issues related to weight so that the individual doesn't have to deal with the many complications of overweight and obesity. Of those, 6.4% are morbidly obese with a BMI of 40 or greater.

The number of overweight and obese individuals rose around the world by more than 145% from 857 million in 1980 to 2.1 billion in 2013 (Global Burden of Disease Study 2013, published in The Lancet).

The Vegetarian Way

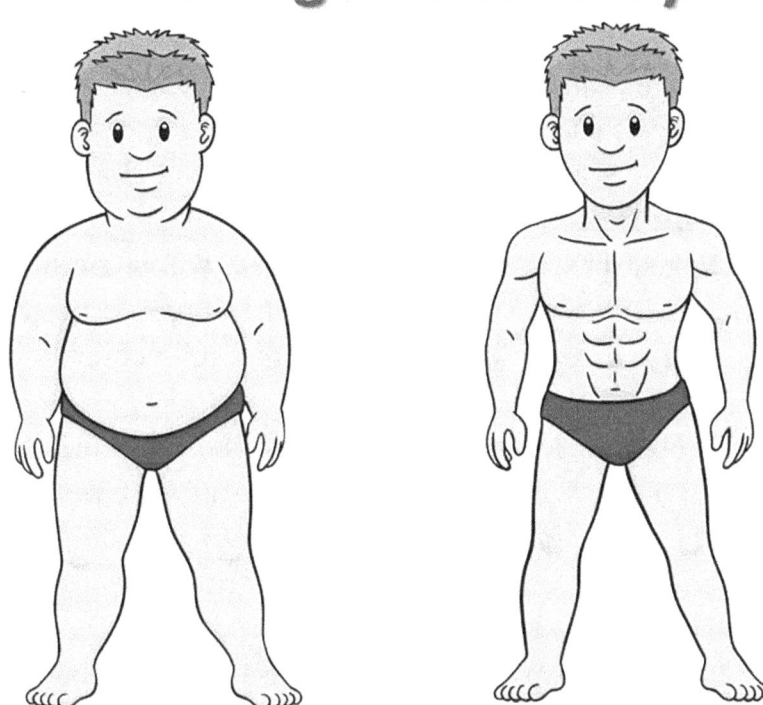

Obesity and overweight are precursors to problems like high blood pressure, cardiovascular problems, type 2 diabetes, and even some types of cancers.

How A Vegetarian Diet Can Help You Lose Weight?

Vegetarian diets are by nature low in calories, especially if you are a vegan. Fruits and vegetables don't have very many calories, so you can eat your fill, not feel hungry, and lose weight at the same time. Fruit generally contain less than 100 calories per serving, while vegetable servings can be far less—as low as 20-50 calories per serving. You can eat a full repertoire of vegetarian food and lose or maintain weight. In fact, vegetarian diets that stick to fruits and vegetables are usually no higher than 1500 calories per day so that you can lose at least one pound a week for every week you stay on such a diet.

What Kind of Vegetarian Diet Works Best for Weight Loss?

Vegetarians who choose to be vegans will eat nothing but fruits, grains, beans, and vegetables, forgoing meat as a protein source as well as the eggs and milk obtained from animals.

Protein is instead obtained from beans and legumes, which are low in fat and calories. Vegan dieters will lose weight more rapidly than other types of eaters simply because there aren't many calories in fruits and vegetables.

For variety, you can buy a vegan cookbook or look up vegan recipes on the internet. These sites and books can supply you with many recipes you can use at home so you won't quickly become bored with just eating raw fruits and vegetables.

Vegetarian Eating to Stay Full

Many overweight people fear going hungry or not feeling satisfied if they adopt a vegetarian diet. This can be fixed by eating several smaller meals several times a day that keep the stomach always working on digesting something and the metabolism going.

When you feel hungry, you have a variety of vegetarian snacks to choose from so that you don't feel deprived of nutrition or foods you like. If you have a large amount of weight to lose, this type of vegetarian diet can be especially helpful because you'll be satisfied with your diet and will lose weight naturally, safely and faster than if, you eat large meals fewer times per day. Small and frequent meals keep your metabolism going so that you burn fat faster and lose more weight.

Using Exercise for Weight Loss

Vegetarians who use the fuel they take in for exercise will lose even more weight. Exercise burns off calories much faster than being sedentary and, if you eat a strictly vegetarian diet you will still have enough energy to exercise for at least a half hour a day.

Choose workouts that get your heart pumping like walking, running, swimming, or dance forms of exercise because they are effective fat burners and also effective for heart health. Vegetarians who also exercise will have low risks for getting cardiovascular diseases such as heart attacks, strokes and peripheral vascular disease. This is because these types of diets are low in cholesterol, which can promote unhealthy plaques on the arteries. The combination of weight loss and a low cholesterol diet makes for a longer lifespan overall. Try it if you have been struggling to lose weight and haven't found the answer yet.

Constipation and Diverticular Disease

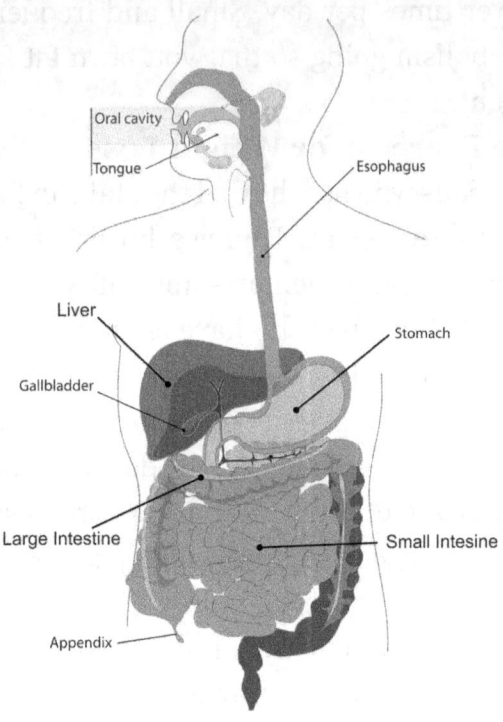

If you find yourself suffering from constipation or were diagnosed with diverticular disease, then consider a vegetarian diet as a way of combating these conditions. When you are constipated, you can stress the lining of the lower digestive tract, causing parts of the lining to form external pouches called diverticuli. These pouches can be medically risky because they collect stool and bacteria and can cause infections such as diverticulitis. The infected diverticuli act similar to appendicitis and can rupture if not treated effectively.

Conquer Diverticular Disease and Constipation with Vegetarianism

Those who follow a vegetarian diet tend to eat a large amount of high fiber foods from beans, lentils, whole fruits, vegetables, and whole grains. The soluble fiber is helpful because it attracts more water into the colon so that stools are softer and pass through the digestive system easier. Researchers have determined that a diet high in fiber from plant based foods support healthy bacteria in the gut. Too many people with constipation or other gastrointestinal complaints are chronically troubled because of unhealthy bacteria in the system.

When you replace unhealthy bacteria with healthy ones, the gut no longer has to deal with the toxins produced by unhealthy bacteria or the gas that these kinds of bacteria make as part of their own metabolism. Your stools should be easier to pass with less gas and bloating.

Vegetarian Foods Actually Reduce Diverticulitis

The food you eat as a vegetarian, particularly those with a lot of fiber, will trap particles of food that are otherwise indigestible and will prevent these particles from blocking the opening to the diverticuli. You lessen your risk of the bacteria becoming stuck in the diverticular pouches infecting the area, causing pain, fever, and inflammation.

Soluble fiber in a vegetarian diet can be found in oats and other grains, and beans. These, fortunately, make up a good portion of a vegetarian diet. Vegetarians, because of their dietary habits, have a more smooth-running digestive tract, which prevents diverticular blockage and subsequent infection that can become systemic and very serious.

Vegetarianism Can Increase the Rate of Stool Passage

Vegetarian diets often contain a great deal of insoluble fiber that comes from the sturdier parts of certain plants, such as broccoli, asparagus, and cauliflower. Insoluble fiber is not digested and therefore is passed through the body as bulk waste. Bulkier stools stimulate the lower digestive system so that the stools move through the colon faster, preventing straining and secondary diverticular disease.

This means that vegetables and fruits in a vegetarian diet should be in their natural, uncooked state, as much as possible. Uncooked vegetables contain solid fiber that will bind with other indigestible plant-derived molecules causing the best rate of stool passage, particularly in the colon, which represents the lower part of the bowels. This means less straining while having a bowel movement, reducing the risk of getting diverticuli and diverticulitis.

Foods to Eat for Digestive Health

As mentioned, eat a vegetarian diet that is in its raw, natural state as much as possible.

Great raw fruits and vegetables include:

- Carrots
- Broccoli
- Kale

- Cauliflower

- Whole apples

- Whole plums

- Whole pears

- Whole peaches

- Citrus fruits

The fiber is in the whole plant so you don't get the benefit from highly cooked vegetarian foods or juices from the fruits. Consider using a blender to make smoothies instead of using a juicer as this method retains the fiber in the raw produce making this type of juice as healthy for you as the entire fruit or vegetable. Look for good vegetarian recipes in a vegetarian cookbook or on the web. You should find recipes that are the most beneficial for your digestive health.

Plant Diets and Fiber

Fiber intake is one of the most important considerations in any type of eating plan, and vegetarian diets are naturally high in this important nutrient. Experts report that Americans typically do not ingest nearly enough fiber in their daily diet.

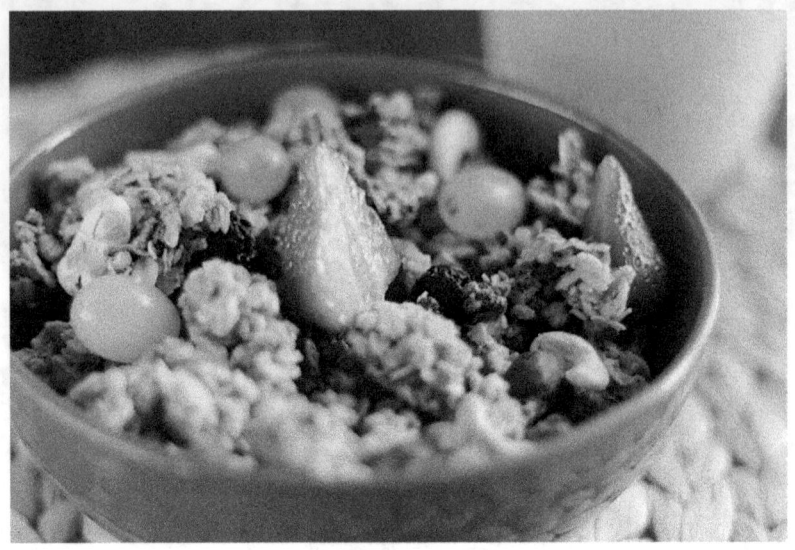

What Is Fiber?

Fiber is dietary material that contains cellulose, lignin, and pectin that resist the action of digestive enzymes.

Two Types of Fiber

- **Soluble fiber** - Soluble fiber is a type that dissolves in water and then forms a gel-like material. Soluble fiber helps to lower blood cholesterol and glucose levels. Oats, beans, apples, carrots, barley, peas, and citrus fruits are good sources of soluble fiber.

- **Insoluble fiber** – Insoluble fiber promotes movement in the digestive track and increases stool bulk and therefore helps to prevent constipation or irregular stools. Good sources of insoluble fiber include wheat bran, nuts, whole-wheat flour, green beans, potatoes, and beans.

Many plant-based foods provide both soluble and insoluble fiber, though the amounts vary from food to food, therefore a highly varied diet that is filled with different plant foods is recommended.

Benefits of High Fiber Diets

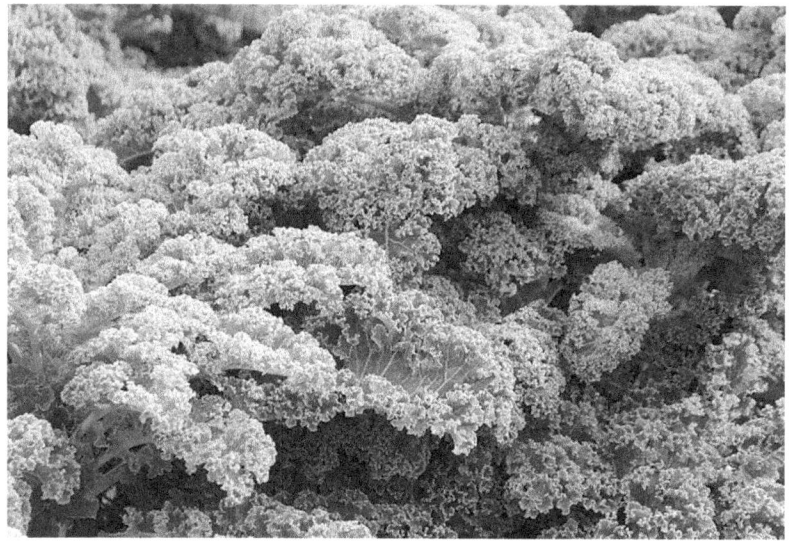

- Fiber fills you up, which results in lower caloric intake and less frequent snacking, supporting healthy weight management.
- Fiber lowers the risk of heart disease.

- Some evidence exists that it may prevent colorectal cancer.
- Fiber helps to lower bad LDL cholesterol, and increases the good HDL cholesterol.
- Fiber lowers the risk of diverticular disease.
- Fiber also lowers the risk of getting gallstones and kidney stones.
- Fiber greatly improves digestive health and maintains bowel health.
- Fiber helps to prevent type 2 diabetes and helps to regulate blood glucose levels in those already diagnosed. Since fiber supports a healthy weight in this way it also helps to manage, reverse and prevent type 2 diabetes.

How Much Fiber Do You Need?

Men age 50 or younger need 38 grams and men age 51 or older need 30 grams. Women age 50 or younger need 25 grams and women age 51 or older need 21 grams

Hypertension

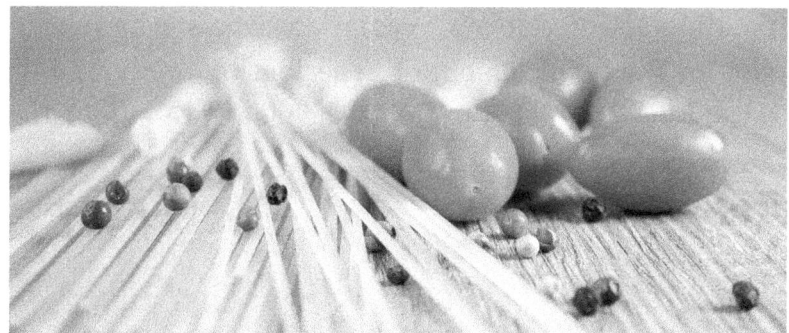

Hypertension is a common condition among people living in countries that eat mostly meat-eating diets. In fact, the prevalence of high blood pressure in men and women residing in the United States is about 30%, and higher in African Americans who have hypertension at a prevalence of about 42%.

Hypertension is the same as "high blood pressure" and is a state of too much pressure in the arteries of the body due to various things, such as a high pulse pressure in the heart or constricted arteries. A blood pressure reading of 140/90 means that the heart pumps at 140 mmHg when it contracts and leaves a residual arterial pressure of 90 mmHg at rest. Hypertension is associated with heart disease, kidney disease, and stroke.

Lowering Blood Pressure with A Vegetarian Diet

Vegetarian diets generally are of a lower calorie count that meat-eating diets, which means that you stand a good chance of losing excess weight and body fat on a vegetarian diet. People who are obese are at a higher risk of high blood pressure and losing weight can reduce blood pressure. Because vegetarians eat mostly fruits and vegetables that are naturally low in calories, vegetarians who start a vegetarian diet for the management of hypertension are bound to eat fewer calories and lose weight. The blood pressure naturally drops as the weight drops.

The Secret of Salt

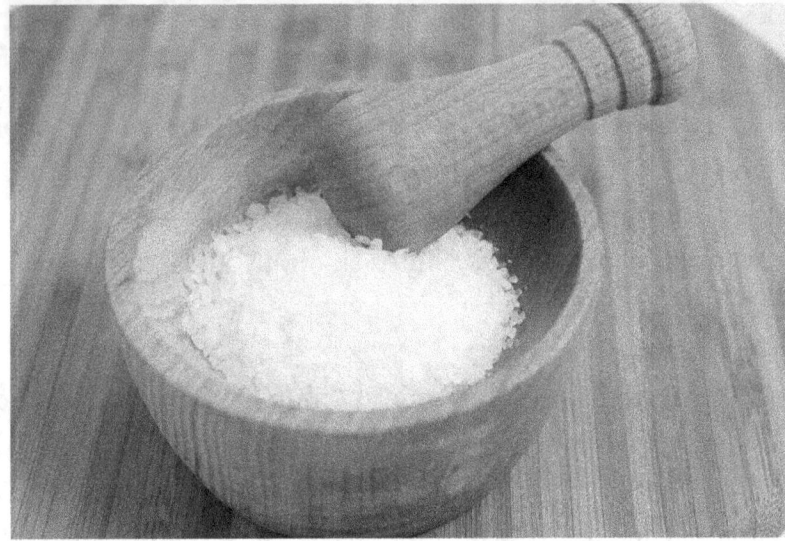

Sodium chloride or table salt contributes to getting high blood pressure, in part because the salt triggers the kidneys to send signals to the blood vessels to raise blood pressure. Vegetarians usually eat plant foods that are naturally unsalted unless they eat a lot of high salt, canned vegetables or add table salt to their food. If a person with hypertension decides to fight it with a vegetarian diet, they must not add a lot of salt to vegetable dishes and must cut out foods that have hidden sources of salt, such as breakfast cereals, bread, salad dressings, cheese, processed soups, bottled sauces, canned foods and food you get at a restaurant.

Foods don't necessarily have to taste salty in order to have a lot of sodium chloride in them. For foods with food labels, you need to look at the sodium content to see how much salt it actually has. Choose low salt alternatives if they are offered at the store.

Minerals and Other Elements of Vegetarian Foods

Almost all vegetables and fruits high in things like magnesium, potassium and other minerals or molecules that are known to be important in halting high blood pressure. Beans especially are high in these compounds. All of these foods are a big part of a vegetarian diet, so there is a natural reduction in blood pressure values when eating them. The combination of low sodium, high potassium content in vegetarian foods makes for low blood pressure readings.

Fighting Hypertension with Vegetarianism

If you find yourself diagnosed with hypertension and don't want to be on medication for the rest of your life, you can begin a vegetarian diet.

You will likely have to be on medication for a period of time until you lose enough weight and allow the positive effects of plant foods to work their magic. Follow your blood pressure at home using a portable blood pressure monitor you can purchase online or at a local pharmacy. If you get consistently lower than acceptable readings, in the range of 100/60 or less, it is time to talk to your doctor about decreasing or stopping the blood pressure medications altogether.

Chronic Kidney Failure

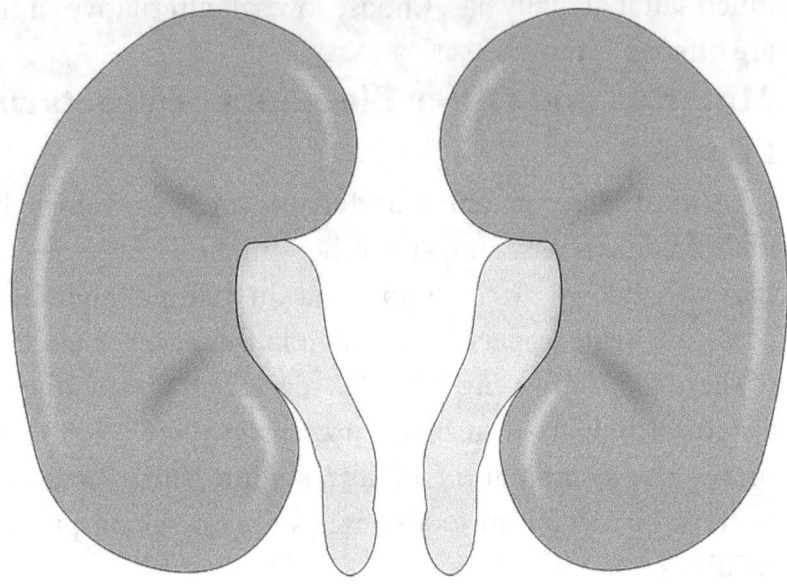

Chronic kidney failure can come from a hereditary kidney disease or from many years suffering from high blood pressure or diabetes. This means that, for those at risk for chronic kidney failure, you could do a lot by reducing the incidence of risk factors. Both high blood pressure and diabetes stress the blood vessels of the kidneys, damaging them so that they send out signals to the body to raise the blood pressure further. Fortunately, both high blood pressure and diabetes can be fought with a vegetarian diet so a change in diet alone can reduce the incidence of chronic kidney disease.

The Effects of Chronic Kidney Disease

Those who suffer from some degree of kidney failure will be less able to filter the blood of toxins and waste products of metabolism. The glomerular filtration rate, which is a measure of the kidney's ability to filter blood, will decrease so that waste products and toxins build up. The kidney responds to the lowered glomerular filtration rate by sending signals that increase the blood pressure. This increase in blood pressure forms a cycle back to causing even worsened kidney failure—a bad cycle that can lead to dialysis or a kidney transplant.

The Vegetarian Diet and Kidney Disease

✓ Vegetarian diets help the kidneys by lowering blood pressure and decreasing the risk of diabetes—known risk factors for chronic kidney failure.

✓ Vegetarian diets are low in sodium, especially if you eat raw vegetables and fruits instead of canned foods. This automatically lowers blood pressure and protects the kidneys.

✓ Vegetarian diets are low in refined sugars in general. It is this reduction in refined sugar that lowers the risk of diabetes, therefore decreasing the risk of secondary chronic kidney failure. It all depends on what kind of vegetarian diet you eat because technically you can eat refined sugars on a vegetarian diet. Most vegetarians don't, however, consume much refined sugar and stay with a diet of healthy fruits, vegetables, grains, beans and legumes. These are naturally low in sugar so that diabetes is less likely and the secondary kidney disease risk diminishes greatly.

Vegetarian Diets Place Less Stress On the Kidneys

The kidneys, even healthy ones, are overly stressed by diets high in protein and sodium. Many years of having to filter these substances through the kidney tubules causes damage to these areas of the kidneys so that the kidneys tend to fail. While it generally takes many years for chronic kidney, failure to show itself in high protein, high sodium diets, this is what meat-eating diets tend to offer. Switching to a low protein, low sodium diet such as a vegetarian diet can relieve the stress on the damaged kidneys, slowing or stopping the progression of chronic kidney failure.

Vegetarians get their protein from dairy products, eggs, and beans, unless they are vegans and don't even take in dairy products or eggs. These foods have the proteins necessary for life but don't have nearly as much protein as is found in a completely meat-eating diet. The kidneys do not have to work as hard for those who eat a vegetarian diet so they last longer without disease.

How to Prevent or Deter Chronic Kidney Disease

If you have a genetic condition like polycystic kidney disease or are at risk for kidney disease by virtue of having high blood pressure or diabetes, it is worth it to see your doctor and a nutritionist who can help you adopt a vegetarian lifestyle that will ultimately help keep kidney disease at bay or can slow the progression of kidney disease you may already have.

Nutrition Concerns

Vegetarian diets are a healthy alternative to the diets consumed by non-vegetarians with their high amounts of saturated fat and cholesterol. However, animal sources of food have certain nutrients that are either not found in a viable form in plants or are not present at all.

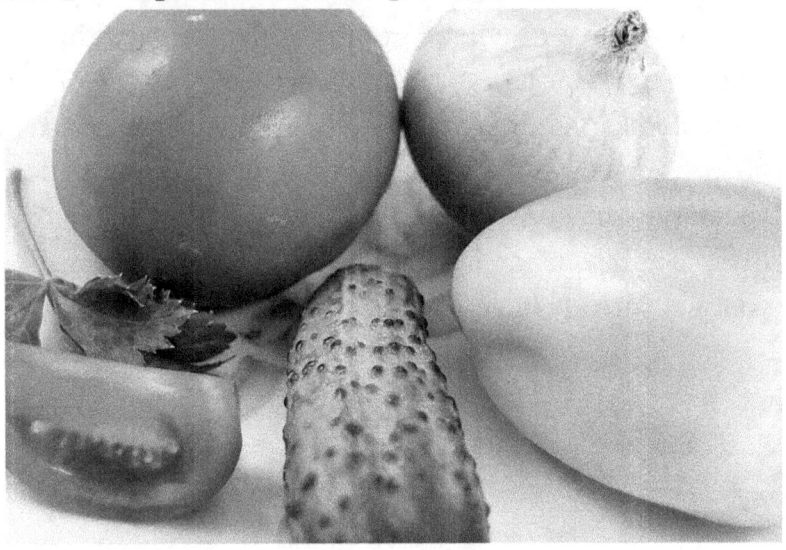

Meat has gotten, to some extent, an undeserved reputation over the years. It's true that the consumption of processed red meat has been linked to heart disease, but then the same could be argued for any processed food including that which is made from white flour and to which sugar is added.

A balanced diet normally includes some form of animal products as prescribed by the Food Pyramid created by the FDA. A balanced diet is one in which all the nutrients needed to keep the body functioning properly are met by a diverse and varied diet.

It is important to understand that a vegetarian diet in in of itself is not a problem. It is very easy for the vegetarian or vegan to eat a balanced diet if appropriate substitutes are used; this fact has been confirmed by the American Diabetes Association and other experts. The problem occurs when vegetarians do not take the time to educate themselves as to the particular nutrients at risk for deficiency, namely those that come from meat and dairy, and how to include proper substitutions for such foods. Here are some of the nutrients at risk for deficiency in the vegetarian diet, and the best plant sources of them.

Protein

Protein is considered the building block of life. Skin, hair, bones, and muscles all need this vital nutrient to do their jobs and to remain strong and healthy. When protein is broken down in the body, it turns into amino acids, which assist with cell growth and cell repair.

Some amino acids, known as essential amino acids, cannot be manufactured by the body they can only be obtained from food. Athletes and children are particularly at risk, since they need a higher level of protein than adults do.

Complete proteins are those that contain all essential amino acids, and are typically found in meat, eggs, and fish. There are several vegan choices. Combining certain foods in meals also creates complete proteins. One such combination is rice and beans.

While meat and eggs are considered some of the highest quality sources of protein, vegans, and vegetarian have available to them a wide variety of plant-based proteins.

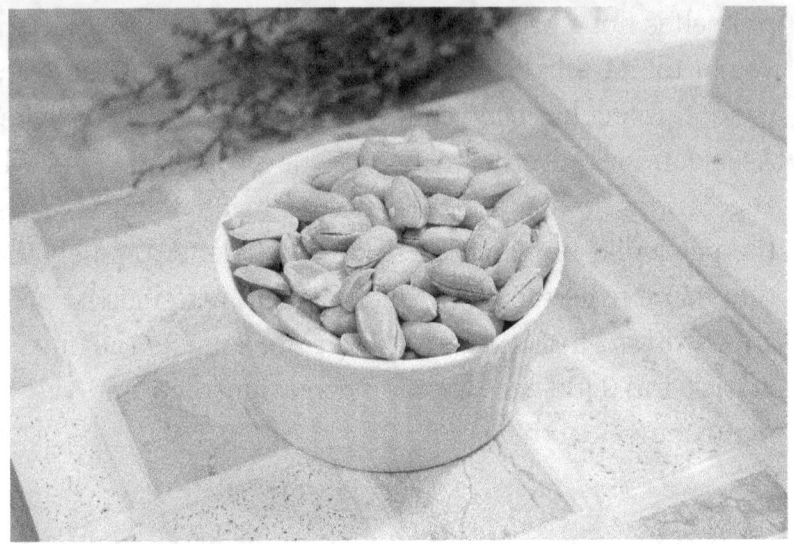

Protein Sources

For vegetarians who eat dairy: milk, Greek yogurt, eggs, cheese.

Complete Vegan Proteins

- Chia: 4 grams per 2 tablespoon serving
- Soy: 10 grams per ½ cup serving (the firmer the tofu the higher the protein content), 15 grams per ½ cup serving (tempeh), 15 grams per ½ cup serving (natto)
- Soybeans: 68 grams per cup
- Mycoprotein (Quorn): 13 grams per ½ cup serving
- Ezekiel Bread (sprouted grain bread): 8 grams per 2 slice serving

- Seitan: 21 grams per 1/3 cup serving
- Quinoa: 8 grams per 1 cup serving, cooked
- Buckwheat: 6 grams per 1 cup serving, cooked
- Hempseed: 10 grams per 2 tablespoon serving

Combinations to Yield Complete Vegan Proteins

- Hummus and Pita: 7 grams per 1 whole-wheat pita with 2 tablespoons of hummus
- Spirulina with Grains or Nuts: 4 grams per 1 tablespoon
- Peanut Butter Sandwich: 15 grams per 2-slice sandwich with 2 tablespoons of peanut butter
- Rice and Beans: 7 grams per 1 cup serving

Other Protein Sources

- **Beans:** navy beans, pinto beans, winged beans, black beans, and others are great protein sources. Chickpeas, lentils, black-eyed peas, and garbanzo beans are too.
- **Nuts and Nut Butters**
- **Seeds:** chia seeds, sunflower seeds, sesame seeds, poppy seeds, pumpkin/squash seeds, hemp, and flaxseeds.

- **Vegetables:** soybean sprouts, lentil sprouts, green peas, corn, sun-dried tomatoes, spinach, kale, bok choy, broccoli, cowpeas, lima beans, Brussel sprouts, mushrooms, artichokes and potatoes.
- **Fruits:** dried apricots, peaches, avocadoes, guava, prunes, dried Zante currants, dried figs, raisins, dates, and passion fruit.
- **Whole grains:** cereals, bread, whole grain pasta, quinoa, oat bran, wheat, buckwheat, couscous, brown rice, and many others.
- **Unsweetened cocoa powder**
- **Veggie burgers**
- **Soy protein prepared foods, such as veggie hot dogs**

Examples of Vegan Protein Substitutes

- Swap bacon and sausage at breakfast for Tofurkey, and soy sausages.
- Swap burgers for veggie burgers, there are many to choose from including those made from soybeans, vegetables, and/or rice.
- Use tofu, tempeh, and seitan in soups, and stews to boost protein.
- Make burgers and meatballs for pasta out of beans, tempeh, lentils, and chickpeas.

Omega-3 Fatty Acids

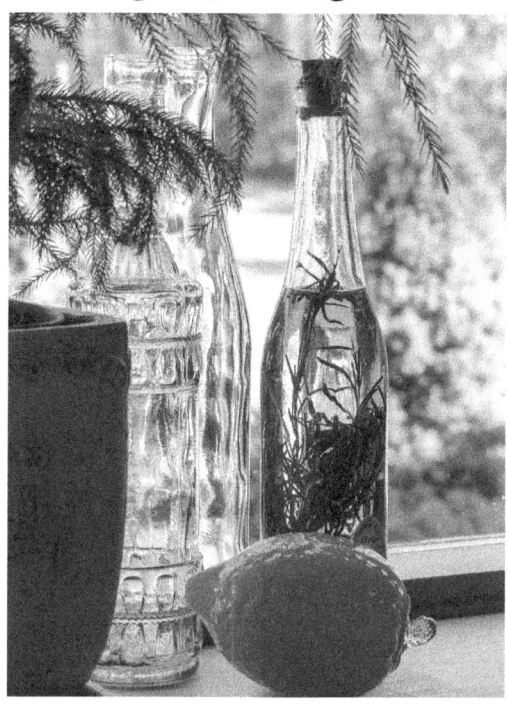

Omega-3s are a part of a group of polyunsaturated fats, which are vital for health. ALA (alpha-linolenic acid) is an omega-3 that the body cannot manufacture on its own, it is obtained from various foods, both animal and plant varieties.

Other omega-3s like DHA (docosahexaenoic acid) and EPA (eicosapentaenoic acid) are the results of our bodies transforming ALA.

Omega-3s are beneficial to the body in several ways:

- They are good for the heart as they lower cholesterol levels, reduce abnormal heartbeats, and lower blood pressure.
- Studies have shown that they may be good for mental health, including memory, learning, and protection against depression and age related problems caused by dementia.
- They support arthritis relief by reducing inflammation in the body.
- They are also good for skin health.

The problem with the vegetarian diet and, particularly the vegan diet is that most plant foods only contain ALA. DHA isn't present in most land plants, except for fermented soy products. Even though DHA and EPA are converted from ALA in the body, there is doubt that humans can get sufficient amounts by this method and so therefore need to consume these nutrients directly from food. Flaxseed is a great source of ALAs but only animal sources, especially fish, contain EPA and DHA.

Our body's absorption of Omega-3s is affected by Omega-6s, which are found in higher quantities in plant foods. Too much Omega-3s can reduce the number of EPAs and DHAs converted from ALAs.

Recommended Intake
Adults need between 1.1 and 1.6 grams of omega-3 fatty acids each day. The vegan diet is most at risk of not getting

sufficient quantities of this nutrient, though supplements are available. It is best to get as much Omega-3s from food as possible.

Vegan Omega 3-Fatty Acids

- Flaxseeds
- Soy products like tofu
- Soybeans
- Navy beans, and kidney beans and mung beans
- Leafy greens: romaine, arugula, spinach and purslane (an edible weed)
- Walnuts and pecans
- Wild rice
- Edamame
- Vegetable oils: corn oil and sunflower oil
- Plant oils: flaxseed oil, linseed oil, canola oil, soybean oil, wheat germ oil and walnut oil
- All cabbages
- Cauliflower, broccoli, bok choy and Brussels sprouts
- Winter squash

Vitamin B12

B12 is an important vitamin and while it does occur in plant foods, it is not useable by humans from these sources. Vitamin B12 does many things for the human body, for example the production of DNA and red blood cells, just to name two.

Typically, the only useable forms found naturally in food come from animal products, such as meat, milk, cheese, and eggs. This means that vegans and vegetarians who do not eat eggs or dairy will risk deficiency of this important nutrient.

B12 Deficiency Can Cause:

- Rapid heartbeat and breathing
- Pale skin
- Sore tongue
- Easy bruising or bleeding
- Stomach upset
- Weight loss
- Diarrhea or constipation
- Cognitive decline and dementia
- Megaloblastic anemia
- Nerve problems
- Fatigue and weakness

Some people absorb this vitamin better than others who may need to take additional amounts, and older people are particularly susceptible to this deficiency.

Vegan Sources of B12

- Fortified non-dairy milks
- Fortified breakfast cereals
- Fortified nutritional yeast

Supplements are also available, consult with a physician before starting use.

Calcium and Vitamin D

Calcium is another nutrient that may be deficient in the vegetarian diet. Dairy foods are the most common sources of calcium. Calcium is contained in plant foods as well, but the presence of oxalic and phytic acids in many calcium rich plant foods, prevents the full absorption of calcium.

Calcium is vital for bone health, especially in growing children, athletes and the aged. Vegans and vegetarians who do not include dairy in their diets are most at risk for deficiency.

Symptoms of Calcium Deficiency Include:

- Increased cramping during PMS
- Weaker bones which results in an increased risk for fractures
- Fingernails that easily break
- Dry skin
- Yellow teeth
- Muscle cramping at nights particularly in the legs

Prolonged deficiency can result in a condition known as Osteoporosis, a progressive bone disease characterized by decreasing bone mass and density that leads to an increased risk of fracture.

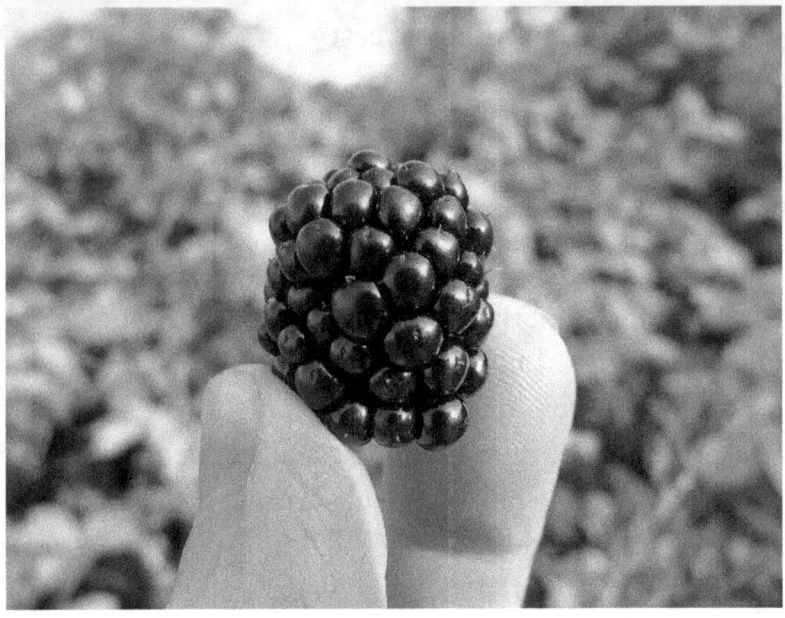

Vegan Calcium Sources

Milk, yogurt, and cheese are traditional sources of calcium; vegans and vegetarians who eliminate dairy can consume these calcium-rich foods to be sure and get enough of this vital mineral.

- Fortified orange juice
- Almonds
- Edamame

- Artichoke, kale, broccoli, bok choy, okra and collard greens
- Tofu
- Blackberries
- Soymilk
- Beans
- Soy beans

Plant foods containing oxalic acids or phytic acids also reduce calcium absorption. Supplementation and calcium-fortified foods will help.

Vitamin D

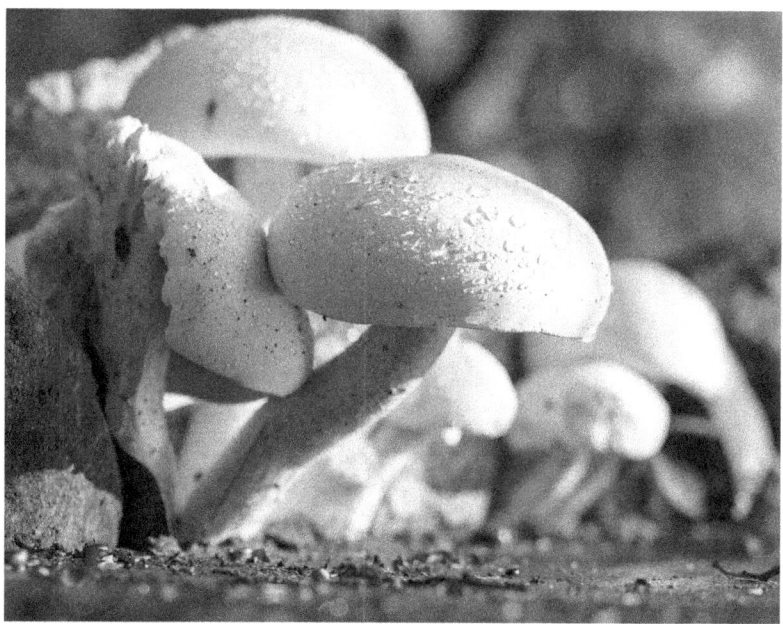

Vitamin D like calcium is necessary for good bone health and works in concert with calcium to help prevent

Osteoporosis. It also helps in the absorption of calcium in the body and plays a role in cardiovascular health. Because it helps the absorption of calcium, it also helps prevent osteoporosis as well as other health problems.

Vitamin D Deficiency Can Cause:

Mild deficiency typically shows no symptoms, but severe deficiency can cause:

- Bones to become weak and brittle, resulting in an increased risk of fractures
- Balance problems due to muscle weakness

Vegan Vitamin D Sources

- Fortified orange juice
- Maitake mushrooms, chanterelle mushrooms (raw) and portabella mushrooms
- Soymilk fortified with vitamin D
- Almond milk fortified with vitamin D
- Fortified soy yogurt
- Fortified ready-to-eat cereals
- Supplements

Lacto-Vegetarian Dairy Vitamin D Sources:

- Milk
- Yogurt
- Eggs

- Swiss cheese

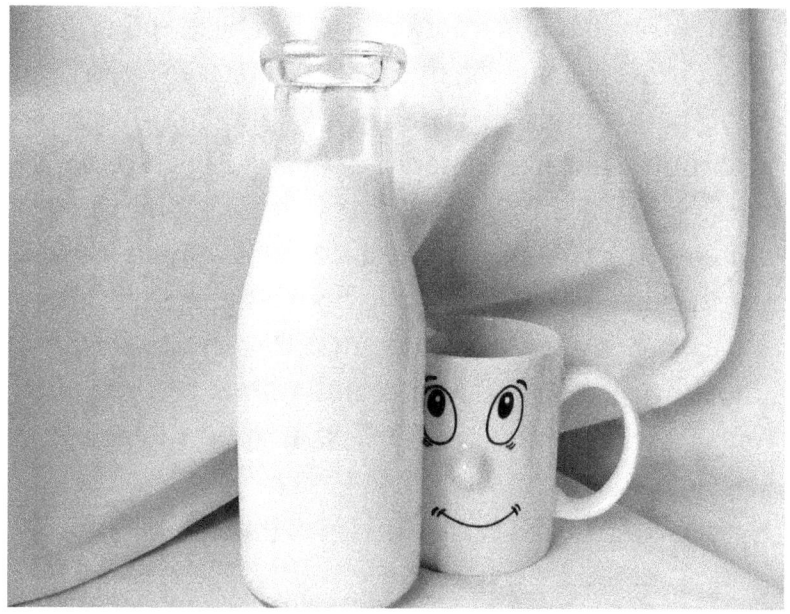

You can easily increase your level of vitamin D by simply spending 10 or 15 minutes a day out in the sunlight.

In regions where exposure to the sun is limited and especially during seasons of the year when the days are shorter, supplementation of vitamin D maybe necessary.

Iron

Iron is necessary for good health. Iron produces hemoglobin, which assists red blood cells with the delivery of oxygen to all parts of the body. A deficiency of this mineral can lead to anemia.

It comes in two forms:

- Heme iron in animal foods

- Nonheme iron in plant foods

Heme iron is much better absorbed by the body that non-heme iron. Because of this, vegetarians tend to store less iron than non-vegetarians do. Vitamin C increases the absorption of this mineral. It also helps overcome the negative effects of the phytonutrients, including phytic acid, tannins, polyphenols, and oxalic acid that inhibit nonheme absorption. Vegetarians can boost their iron intake by increasing their intake of vitamin C with citrus fruits, and colored vegetables, like red and yellow bell peppers and tomatoes. Broccoli, strawberries, and red cabbage are also excellent sources of vitamin C.

Symptoms of Iron Deficiency

- Feelings of tiredness combined with irritability, weakness, and inability to focus due to loss of oxygen delivery to the tissues.
- Headaches that result from swelling of the arteries in the brain that is not receiving ample oxygen can also occur.
- Cravings for ice by women are sometimes experienced.
- Anxiety triggered by lack of oxygen to the nervous system.
- Hair loss occurs in cases of extreme anemia, since the body is now reserving oxygen for more important functions.

- Shortness of breath can occur due to low oxygen levels, so that normal exercise or slight exertion that was easily managed before now causes breathlessness.

Vegetarians and vegans are at a great risk for iron deficiency since much of the human diet derives this nutrient from red meat. Those who follow a plant based need to take care and include plant sources of iron or use a supplement as necessary.

Vegan Sources of Iron

Dried fruit, broccoli, soybeans, and legumes are all great sources of iron. Supplements are available.

Zinc

Zinc is a mineral that contributes to immune system health. The typical diet obtains this mineral from shellfish, cheese, and red meat.

Zinc Deficiency Can Cause:

- A weak immune system
- Wounds that are slow to heal
- A loss of appetite
- Hair loss
- Dermatitis

Phytates found in some plant foods can impair the absorption of zinc increasing the need for the mineral in vegans. There are ways of maximizing the absorption of this mineral by the strict vegetarian or vegan, they include:

- Preparing grains by soaking before cooking
- Consuming sprouted legumes
- Eating fermented foods
- Consuming toasted nuts and seeds

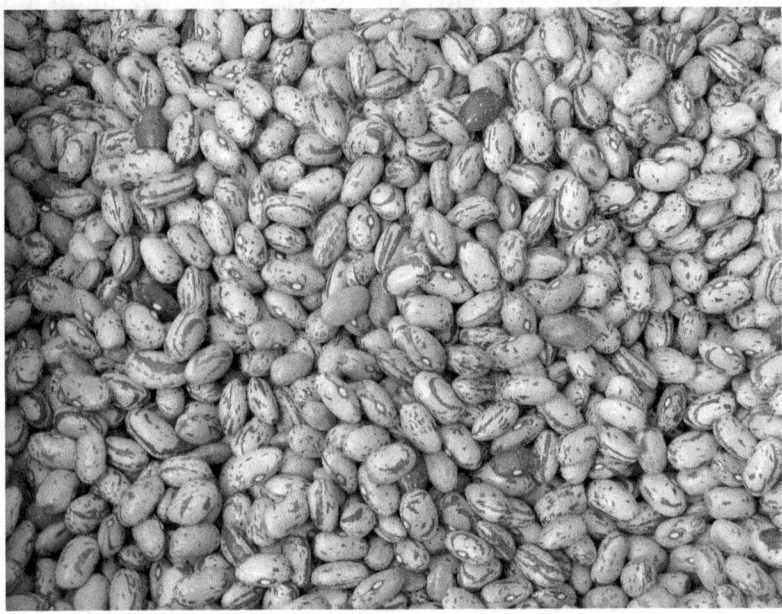

Vegan Zinc Sources:

For those who include dairy, cheese is a good source of zinc.

- Whole grains
- Beans
- Mushrooms

- Nuts
- Soy products
- Wheat germ
- Supplements

Bottom Line

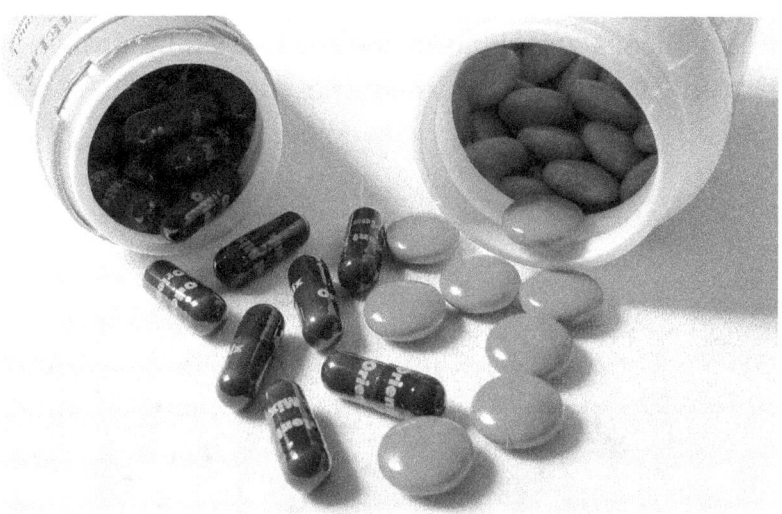

A vegetarian diet can be very healthy when those nutrients at risk for deficiency are addressed and proper vegan sources are added. The vegan needs to be even more watchful than other types of vegetarians, since they follow the most restrictive type of diet.

Consulting with a dietician can help with planning a well-balanced plant diet that will ensure the inclusion of all the vital nutrients the body needs and address any possible need for supplements.

What You Can Eat on a

Vegetarian Diet

There are plenty of food choices for vegetarians and vegans to enjoy. There are also hundreds of vegetarian recipe books and thousands of recipes online from a wide variety of cultures and countries so you need never get bored.

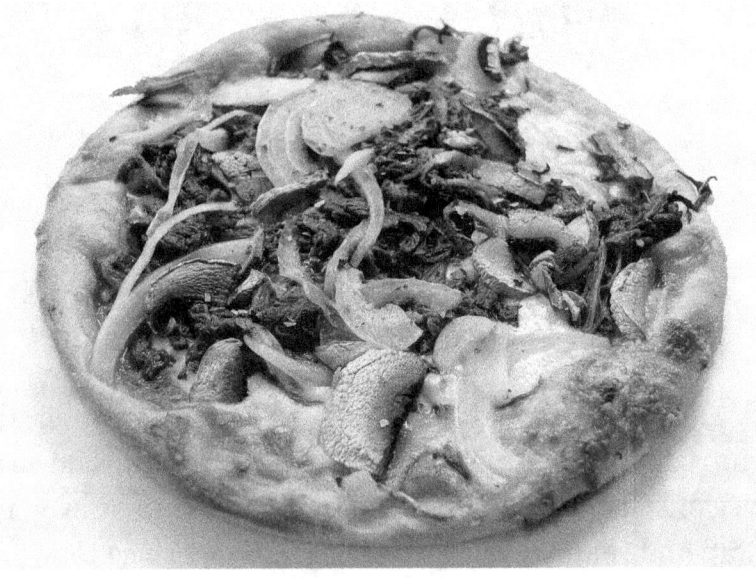

Vegetarians and Vegans Enjoy:

- Tofu, tempeh, and other soy proteins that mimic meat and poultry and can be used as substitutes for such in various recipes
- Beans and lentils
- Seeds and nuts
- All vegetables and fruits
- Whole grains, including bread, cereals, rice and pasta
- Oils from plant seeds, like olive, safflower, canola, soybean, corn and grapeseed
- Dairy for those who choose to include it, including eggs, milk, yogurt and cheese
- There are also many vegetarian soy products, like hot dogs, bacon, sausage, veggie burgers, and chicken nuggets. The many great choices of meat substitutes can still allow you to enjoy your favorite dishes
- Baked goods in moderation

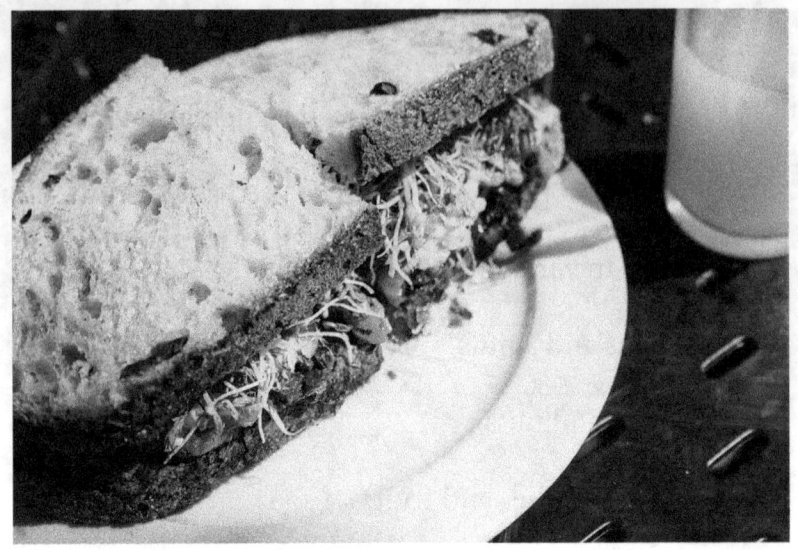

Your New Food Groups

You might think that you're limited to a few fruits and veggies. You're not. We're going to look at 10 different food groups, starting with nuts.

Nuts

Nuts are packed with fiber and protein. They're super filling, which makes them great as a snack. However, you can also use nuts for protein drinks. You can add them to salads and veggie wraps. You can make a delicious pesto sauce with pistachios (or pine nuts) and a little olive oil and parmesan. If you aren't eating dairy, then you can skip the cheese. Add some garlic and enjoy with pasta.

Nuts to consider adding to your pantry include:

- Almonds
- Hazelnuts

- Pistachios
- Walnuts
- Pecans
- Macadamia
- Brazil
- Peanuts (they're actually a legume or bean, but we'll put them here)

Seeds

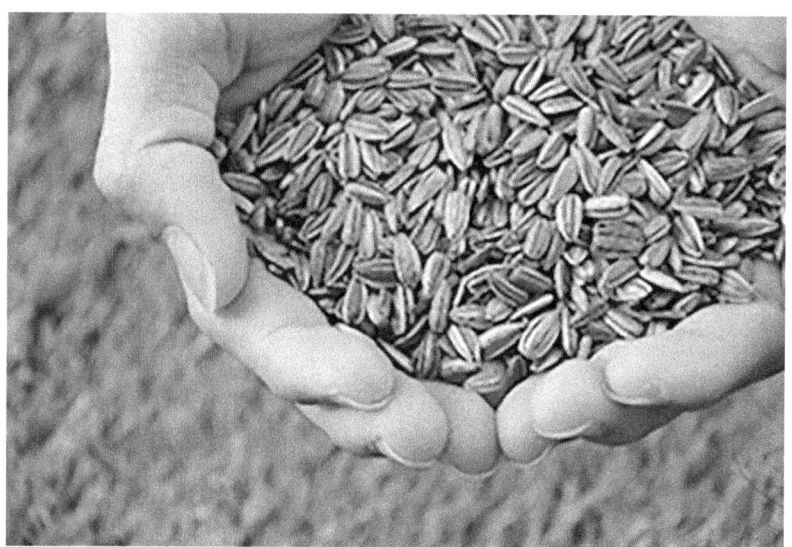

When you think about seeds your thoughts probably head straight for the sunflower seed. Sure, that's a great one, but there are also many others. Again, they're super high in both fiber and protein, which means they leave you feeling full and satisfied. And both seeds and nuts have good plant-based fats in them.

Seeds to consider include:

- Sunflower
- Chia
- Quinoa (it's often considered a grain because of how it's cooked, but it's a seed)
- Flax seeds
- Hemp seeds

Both flax and hemp are often used to make protein powders, and you can find them in the health food store. Seeds are great for adding to salads. Quinoa is extremely versatile and can be made into a meal. You can sauté veggies and serve them on a bed of quinoa. You won't feel deprived, it's delicious. Chia is amazing in granola mixes and you can add it to your yogurt (soy yogurt or dairy depending on your approach.)

Whole Grains

This list is extensive. Grains will likely take up a good amount of your plate when you're meal planning. They're also quite versatile. You can make a cold quinoa salad for example, or you can enjoy faro in a garlic sauce. The sky is the limit. So here is a good list of your whole grain options:

- Amaranth

- Barley
- Brown Rice
- Buckwheat
- Bulgur (Cracked Wheat)
- Faro
- Kamut
- Millet
- Oats
- Rye
- Sorghum
- Spelt
- Teff
- Triticale
- Barley
- Wheat Berries

Brown rice is on the list; you can also have white rice. People often steer clear of this because its starchiness. It's kind of like choosing a piece of white bread over a piece of whole wheat bread. The white bread is okay, but not as good for you as the whole wheat bread. So let's take a look at starchiness next and talk about those amazing starchy vegetables.

Starchy Veggies

Starchy veggies are things like corn, sweet potatoes, yams, and potatoes. They are high on the glycemic index and have more glucose than other vegetables. They're also not as high in protein as most other options. However, as you transition to a plant-based diet they can really be useful.

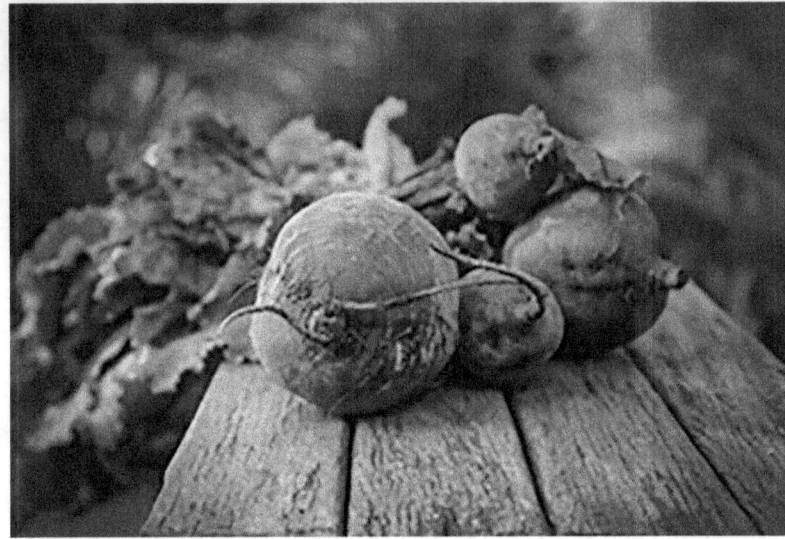

Sweet potatoes and yams are particularly useful. They're a little lower than corn and potatoes on the glycemic index. They taste great for breakfast, lunch, or dinner, and they make a great snack. You can even slice them thin and make chips. If you really need help getting through cravings, and if you're hungry, then they are a nice treat. Here are a few more starchy veggies to consider:

- Beans
- Beets
- Carrots
- Green Peas
- Parsnips

- Taro
- Squash: winter, butternut squash, or pumpkin

Non-Starchy Veggies

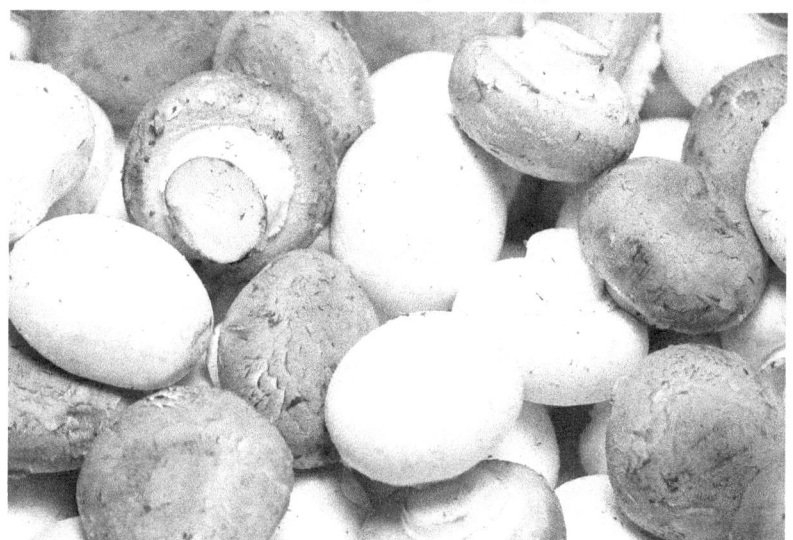

The fun begins. You know, if you stand in the center of your grocer's produce section, there is a seemingly endless variety of vegetables. From peppers and tomatoes to spinach and collards, you have a ton of choice. And of course you can steam, sauté, puree, or eat them raw. You can make sauces from them. Get creative. You can make noodles from a lot of vegetables. Try it with zucchini!

And here's a short list of some options to enjoy:

- Artichoke

- Asparagus
- Avocado
- Bok Choy
- Broccoli
- Brussels sprouts
- Cabbage (red, green, Chinese)
- Cauliflower
- Celery
- Cucumber
- Eggplant
- Fennel
- Green beans (There are other beans too, white, long, French etc....)
- Greens (collard, beet greens, dandelion, mustard, kale, turnip)
- Hearts of palm
- Jicama
- Leeks
- Lettuce
- Mushrooms
- Okra
- Peas (sugar snap, snow and good old green peas)
- Peppers (red, green, yellow, jalapeno, orange)
- Radishes

- Spinach
- Sprouts
- Swiss chard
- Watercress
- Zucchini

Fruits

Fruits will play a role in your plant-based diet. There are literally hundreds of different fruits to try, so listing them would take too much time. Think about berries, pit fruits, dried fruits, tropical fruits and so on. Add fruit to yogurt, puree, or make an awesome morning smoothie. Spread some cream cheese on a pizza crust, top with fruit, and enjoy a dessert pizza.

Beans

Like fruit, there are literally hundreds of different types of beans. Beans have protein and fiber, like nuts. And beans combined with rice makes a complete protein. This is important for strict vegans who are unable to get complete proteins any other way.

Complete proteins are found in animal products. They're important to your health at the cellular level. They're also delicious and versatile. You can puree them to make spreads, dips and sauces. For example, chickpeas are the base of hummus. Lentils are amazing, and soybeans can be eaten steamed with a little salt.

Fats and Oils

Most oils are plant-based. Canola oil, olive oil, coconut oil, and avocado oil too. They can be a tasty and healthy alternative to butter, lard, and bacon fat. There are also "butter" substitutes that are plant-based. Don't avoid fats and oils.

When they're plant-based they're good for you. They also aid in digestion, cellular metabolism, and your immune system. Use plant-based fats and oils in baking, in your sautés, and any other recipe.

Dairy Alternatives

Dairy is one element of a plant-based diet that many people struggle with. Getting rid of cheese and milk can be difficult. However, there are a large number of great alternatives. Soy has been a dairy alternative for a while. Soy milk, soy cheese, and soy ice cream are all options. You can even find chocolate soy milk.

Coconut milk, hemp milk, almond milk, and even rice and cashew milk are all options too. And you can find ice cream made from those ingredients as well. Keep tasting and find one that you like. You can use them in baking, on cereal, and to enjoy on their own.

Meat Alternatives

Meat alternatives get a bad rap. Tofu, tempeh, and veggie burgers are all options. There are burgers made from beans and grains. Quinoa, as mentioned earlier, is a seed that is rich in protein. If you find yourself craving meat, and that can happen, consider trying a meat alternative. Add tofu to a stir fry or fry it until it's crisp. Try different veggie burgers until you find a flavor and consistency that you enjoy.

Now that we have a long list of plant-based foods, so much so that your head may be spinning, it's time to talk about the next step. Choosing your approach – how are you going to embrace a plant-based diet?

Easy Plant Food Swaps

As previously mentioned, you can still enjoy your favorite dishes but without the meat. The good news is that human imagination knows no bounds in being able to duplicate recipes and eatery favorites without the meat, so you can enjoy your new meatless lifestyle without feeling deprived. Pretty much anything you used to eat can be duplicated with plant-based ingredients, including meatballs, and burgers.

Here are some great substitutions for meat in your favorite dishes:

Pizza - The sausage on pizza can be replaced with soy sausage or simply topped with vegetables.

Burgers - Hamburgers can be made with veggie burgers instead of beef, or even enjoyed with a pile of tomatoes, lettuce, onions, and pickles on a fresh baked bun. Eggplant makes a wonderful substitute for beef patties in burgers, as do potatoes, and Portobello mushrooms.

Tacos - Substitute beef in tacos with black beans.

Tofu - Tofu is a protein that is made from soybeans, virtually any recipe that calls for meat can be made with this plant-based protein. Tofu can be used to create tofu nuggets, or used in chunks in stir-fry to replace steak or chicken. Tofu is very good at absorbing flavors of any kind, such as sauces and marinades. Tofu can be cubed, just like chicken or steak for a weekend BBQ kabob. Tofu can also be scrambled to replace eggs. It works great in Thai, Italian, and curry dishes.

Tempeh - Tempeh is also made from soybeans but is much firmer than tofu and so it can be used to make vegan sandwiches like the Rueben or pulled pork. Tempeh has a flaky texture so it's great for crab cakes or vegan fish sticks. You can also grind tempeh to make meatballs or filling for tacos. The possibilities and recipes available are limitless.

TVP - TVP (Textured Vegetable Protein) is a vegetable protein made from soy, can be obtained in all shapes and sizes, and makes a great replacement for any cut of meat, including ground beef. Look for specific recipes online to create tasty vegan dishes with this diverse plant-based protein.

Seitan - Seitan is another great meat substitute made from wheat gluten. Seitan takes on flavors really well and makes a great replacement for pork, chicken, and beef. Recipes like Seitan steak with red wine sauce can quickly make you forget top sirloin. Seitan cacciatore turns an old Italian favorite vegan.

Mushrooms - Mushrooms are very meaty, rich and have an earthy flavor that makes them a perfect beef replacement. In fact, you can build an entire main dish out of a large Portobello mushroom. They can be stuffed with any type of vegetables, such as peppers, spinach, onions, zucchini, and tomatoes and baked. If you eat dairy as part of your plan, melt mozzarella or cheddar cheese over them for added goodness. Stuff them with nuts like pecans for a wonderful rich nutty flavor. They can be grilled with garlic and vegan butter and piled over a hot French or whole grain roll to make a filling and tasty sandwich.

Lentils - Lentils make great meat substitutes. Lentils are healthy, loaded with nutrients, a quality protein, and are hardy enough to replace meat in many dishes. They are cheap and come in a wide variety and colors, including, red, yellow, brown, and green. They can be used in chili, burgers, soups, stews, Shepherd's pie, and meatballs for pasta dishes.

Beans- Beans are fantastic sources of protein and make great meat replacements in vegan diets. Choose from the very inexpensive and filling varieties, such as kidney, black, pinto, or aduki beans along with black-eyed and chickpeas, just to name just a few. Mung beans provide the added benefit of Omega-3 fatty acids.

Beans make for hearty soups, stews, and chilies. Chickpeas make a great tuna salad, and black beans go great in tacos and chili instead of beef. Hummus, which is made from chickpeas, makes a great substitute for mayonnaise on burgers and sandwiches. There are endless varieties of bean salads that add color and flavor to a cool summer dish.

Vegetables - Roasted vegetables can serve as a main dish, and when they are flavored correctly can really wow your taste buds. Mushrooms, eggplant, beets, and potatoes both white and sweet can be made the stars of any meal, including breakfast, lunch, and dinner. With the use of herbs, spices, and sauces like Balsamic vinegar and soy sauce the possibilities become endless in using hearty vegetables to create vegan meals.

Imitation Crab - Thankfully, imitation crab is vegan and tastes yummy, use it for seafood salad, crab cakes, stir-fry, soups or simply to munch on for a midday snack.

Strong Flavors - Replacing strong flavored meats, such as bacon can be achieved in various ways. Tempeh bacon is available, but may not be easy to find in all areas of the country. Using hickory smoked salt or smoked paprika are good alternatives. Other spices, such as chipotle pepper adds a nice smoky flavor to vegan dishes. Liquid smoke can be found in the sauce aisle of your supermarket and a little goes a long way to adding a nice smoky flavor to any dish.

Pumpkin - This Halloween superstar makes for a great meat alternative, especially when it's pureed and added to marinara sauce for pasta dishes.

Okara - Okara is made from soy pulp and contains loads of protein and fiber. It makes a great meat replacement in stews, omelets, and soups. It also makes fantastic crab cakes.

Quinoa – Nature's super food, quinoa is a complete source of protein and also provides you with folic acid, and magnesium. Quinoa is oh so versatile that you will wonder how you ever ate without it. It makes for hearty salads, side dishes, and pilafs and can be baked in patty form for a truly gourmet vegan burger.

Sloppy Joes - How about sloppy Joes made with tofu? When made with a zesty and flavorful sauce, you will never miss the beef, promise!

Buy It Premade - There are also packaged soy protein vegan copies of meat favorites, including tempeh bacon, breakfast sausages, burgers, hot dogs, chicken nuggets, chicken marsala, chicken picatta, pizza, corn dogs and many more. These foods offer nutrition, flavor, and convenience.

The above is really just a shortlist to get you started. Hundreds if not thousands of recipes exist online and in cookbooks for using all the above foods and others in vegan cooking to create tasty and healthy dishes that are loaded with flavor. With so many delicious options, memories of meat will quickly fade away.

Syrups for Honey

Honey is made by bees. Maple and agave syrups are plant-based sweeteners. Date syrup and pure vegetable purees can also effectively replace honey. As with all other plant-based swaps, make sure you are choosing natural, organic, preservative-free products.

Swap Greens for Flour Wraps

Wraps usually begin with a large, flat, circular grain or flour-based outer shell. You place your meat, fish, vegetables, condiments and other toppings on this base, and then "wrap" the outer layer over the inner ingredients, tucking the ends over to make a spill-proof, cylindrical, handheld alternative to a sandwich.

The problem with many wrap exteriors is that they often contain animal and dairy byproducts. Greens with large leaves, like cabbage, butter lettuce, kale and collard greens, make healthy plant-based alternatives to processed wraps. You wrap your ingredients in a large leaf of those vegetables. The wonderful anticancer compounds and antioxidants found in leafy greens are just extra benefits.

In with the Cauliflower...

...for wraps, pizza crust, rice, couscous, potatoes

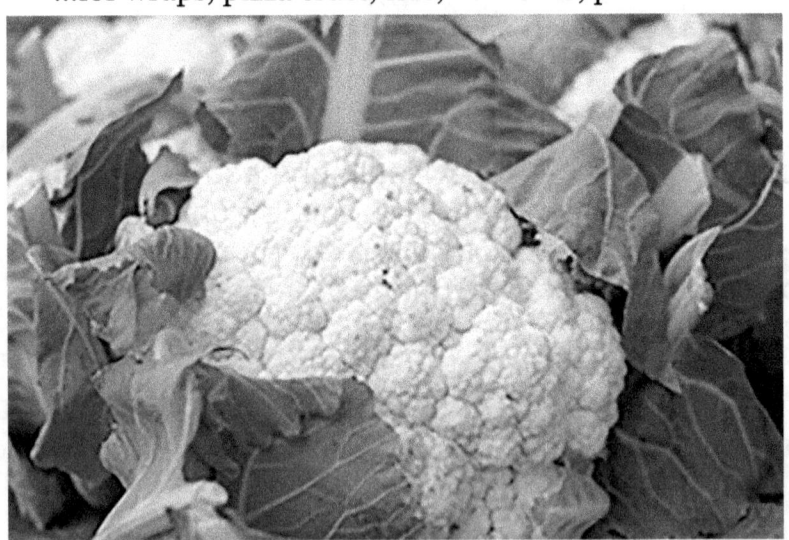

You just discovered how large vegetable leaves

make excellent wrapping material. Did you know you can use cauliflower the same way? Natural, organic cauliflower can be ground down into powdered form using a food processor or food chopper. It can then be used as a base for breads and wraps. It is also the perfect alternative too unhealthy, processed, preservative-filled and dairy-based pizza crusts.

Cauliflower additionally makes the perfect alternative to rice or couscous. Use a food chopper, and stop when the cauliflower has been ground down to the size of rice grains. Sauté in a little coconut oil in a pan for a tasty and super-healthy rice alternative. The versatile cauliflower is not done yet. You can also swap it into a multitude of dishes were potatoes are traditionally used. The first time you taste mashed cauliflower instead of mashed potatoes, you will probably be shocked by the similarity in texture and taste.

One good book to help you realize the true versatility of cauliflower in a plant-based approach to nutrition is "Cauliflower Cookbook: Top 50 Most Delicious Cauliflower Recipes (Superfood Recipes Book 17)", available on Amazon for immediate download, currently just $0.99.

Ditch the Dairy for Nondairy Options

Swap out dairy milk for soy or almond milk. When you were growing up, your parents probably told you to drink a lot of whole milk. Do not blame them for giving you the wrong information. They were simply passing on what they were told by their parents, and in many cases, the nutrition and food authorities in the country where they were raised. We now know that dairy causes constipation and gas, bloating and diarrhea, and has been linked to higher rates of obesity and chronic conditions like diabetes and some cancers.

That is why it is a good idea to make a plant-based swap of soy or almond milk for dairy milk. Just make sure your nondairy food product is free from carrageenan. That substance has been linked to digestive problems, from mild too severe. Vegan cheeses and yogurts also effectively replace their traditional dairy-based counterparts.

Whole Wheat or Nut Flour Instead of White Flour

White flour is not only devoid of almost all nutrition, it has also has had its nutrients replaced by unhealthy chemicals, preservatives and byproducts. White flour lasts longer on grocery store shelves when all is nutrients have been taken out.

Even when you see a sign that says "enriched" on a white flour product, that enrichment occurs only after all the natural goodness has been removed. Replacing white flour with whole wheat or nut flours makes for a healthier, plant-based choice. You can also opt for a black bean purée instead of white flour.

Plant-Based Sugar Replacements

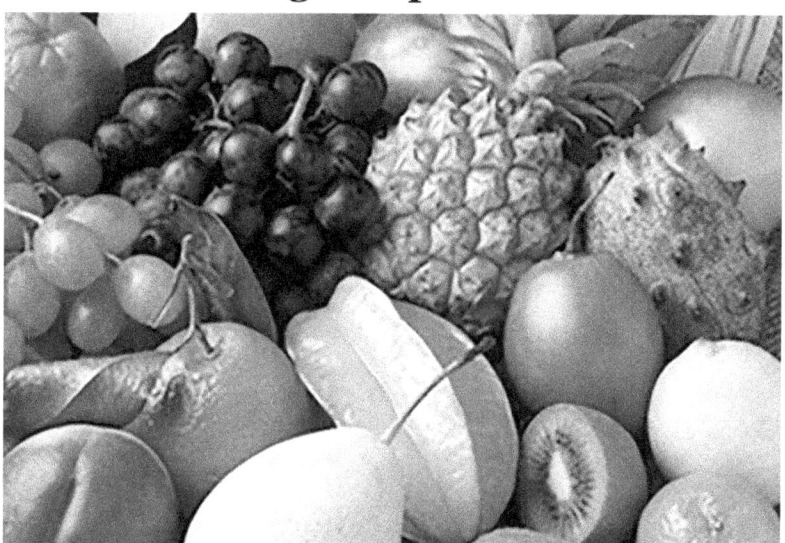

Sugar has been linked to diabetes, overweight, obesity, cancer and a long list of health problems. This can be avoided. There are wonderful natural sweeteners. They can take the place of refined, processed sugar. Every cup of sugar that you replace with a cup of unsweetened applesauce cuts more than 600 calories from your waistline. Just be sure you read your food labels, and avoid highly processed varieties.

Vanilla extract is an often overlooked sugar replacement. You can replace up to half the sugar in any recipe with vanilla extract without dramatically changing the flavor or taste. For every cup of sugar replaced you eliminate 400 calories. In baked goods and other recipes, you can replace 1 cup of sugar with 1 teaspoon of vanilla extract + 1/2 cup of sugar.

The Stevia plant is 300 times sweeter than sugar. Another eyebrow-raising fact is that this natural plant, as sweet as it is, delivers 0 calories! For each cup of sugar in a recipe, replace with 1 teaspoon of liquid Stevia or 2 tablespoons of Stevia powder. Do not be confused by the similarly marketed Truvia, which claims to have Stevia in it. There is very little Stevia contained in Truvia.

Use an Avocado or Banana Purée Instead of Butter

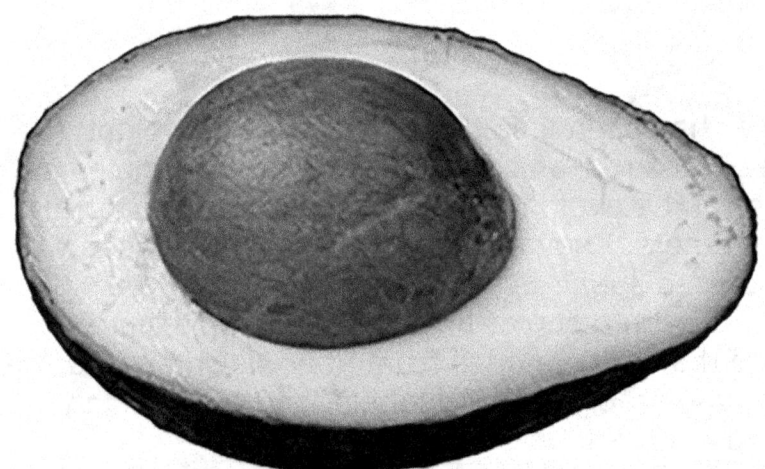

Though it may not seem possible, you can replace butter with plants. A purée made from bananas or avocados contains up to 5 times fewer fat grams, as well as 400% fewer calories, then traditional butter. This swap can be used in all types of recipes, from baked goods to casseroles and anywhere else your recipe requires butter. Make an even swap, 1 cup of butter for 1 cup of banana or avocado purée. Be aware that this usually reduces cooking time up to 25%.

Swap Veggie-Based Patties for Beef Burgers

The hamburger - a bun, the condiments and toppings of your choice, and at least one patty of ground meat, usually beef. Yummy, versatile and full of protein, the hamburger can be pan-fried, flame-broiled or barbecued. Since immigrants from Hamburg, Germany introduced a broiled beef and onion beef burger patty to Ohio in the early 1800's, the hamburger has been a commonplace and inexpensive item at American dinner tables.

Worldwide as well, the hamburger is a popular meat-based protein source. Unfortunately, studies in recent years have pointed to animal-based proteins as directly linked too higher than average cancer rates. The good news? That elevated cancer risk can be prevented, and cancer even reversed, with a plant-based diet.

Thanks to veggie-loving burger worshippers, you can still get that beefy burger taste ... with a plant-versus-beef patty. Make the following veggie-for-beef swaps for some surprisingly great tasting plant burgers.

- Black beans
- Kidney beans
- Mixed vegetables

- Tofu
- Portobello mushrooms
- Potatoes
- Eggplant

There are also some great-tasting, healthy pre-made veggie burgers. The Huffington Post conducted a taste test, and of the dozens of frozen veggie burgers tested, here are the top 5 for taste.

- Dr. Praeger's Kale Veggie Burger
- Gardein Ultimate Beefless Burger
- Hilary's Eat Well World's Best Veggie Burger
- Gardenburger Original Veggie Burger
- Morningstar Garden Veggie Patty

Choose Fruits Over Fruit Juice

Manufactured, processed fruit juices are always marketed as healthy. In most cases, however, you are just looking at sugar in disguise. Fruit juices will many times claim that they have fiber and more Omega 3s or other healthy nutrients added. Unfortunately, often times that fiber is synthetic and extremely hard to digest.

This causes bloating and digestive problems, and sugar can lead too overweight, obesity, cancer and heart problems. Always choose to make your own juice at home, using natural, fresh, organic fruits. Eating real fruits can help you lose weight and manage a healthy body weight, as natural fruit is full of fiber, vitamins and minerals which make you feel full quickly, and limit your calorie intake.

Go with Fresh Veggies Over Frozen

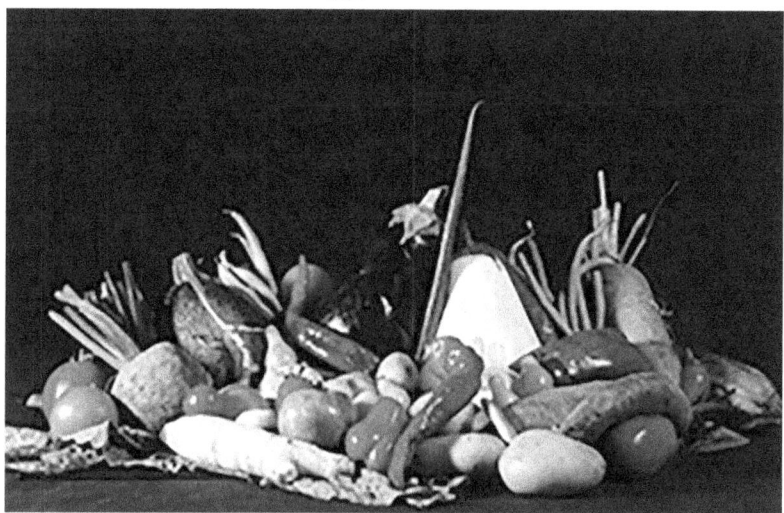

Anytime you can eat fresh plants over frozen, canned, or processed alternatives, you are doing your body a favor. Some frozen meals make boastful health claims. Even so, they are usually cram-packed full of extremely high levels of sodium, preservatives and man-made chemicals you do not need in your body. It takes longer to prepare a meal using natural, fresh vegetables than it does heating up their frozen counterparts. However, this is the right move every time as far as your health is concerned.

Beans Nature's Perfect Plant

Food

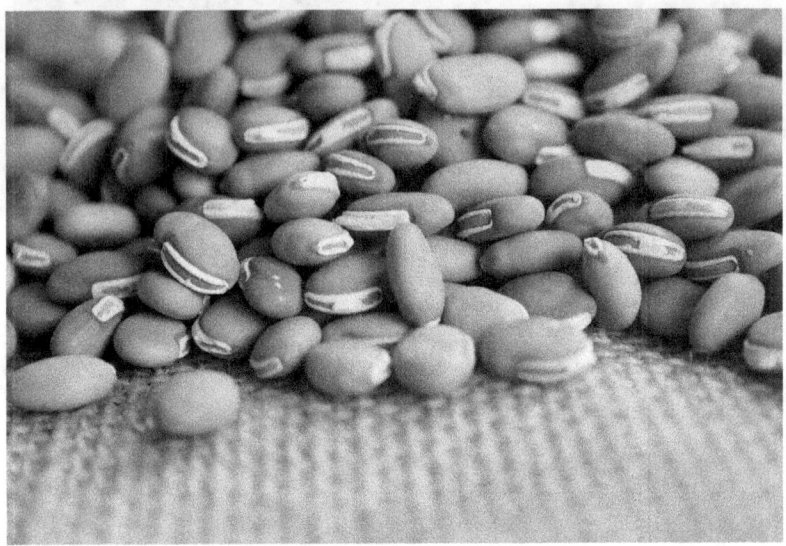

Bean is a common name for large seeds, which are used for human and animal food. Beans are one of the longest-cultivated plants and have been an important source of protein since the second millennium BCE.

Beans have a **significant amount of both fiber and soluble fiber**, and one cup of cooked beans can provide between nine and thirteen grams of fiber.

As well as being **high in protein**, beans are also high in **complex carbohydrates, folate, and iron**.

Another lesser known fact is that either some beans are **exceptionally high in antioxidants**, in fact, even higher than blueberries or cranberries are.

Beans are not referred to as either a fruit or a vegetable and, in fact, are often classified as legumes. Legumes also refer to peas, lentils, and peanuts.

Beans are available in dried forms as well as canned, and both offer you high levels of nutritional value, with the canned options simply being more convenient.

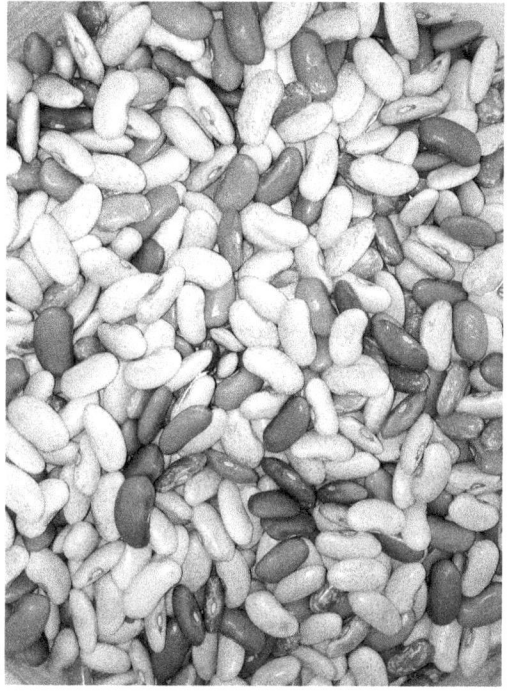

Currently, **dietary guidelines are recommending that we consume three cups of beans a week**. There are many reasons why beans are so good for you.

Key Nutrients in Beans

Beans are high in protein, fiber, iron, folate, and antioxidants. Beans are also high in magnesium, B vitamins, copper, zinc, and potassium, but what are these nutrients and why are they important?

Protein

Protein is essential throughout your entire body. Your body uses protein to make enzymes, hormones and to build and repair tissues.

Protein is also essential for the creation of bones, muscles, cartilage, skin, hair, nails, and blood.

A 1 cup serving of any bean will give anyone at least 20% of daily-recommended protein intake.

Pinto, kidney, adzuki, garbanzo, black, navy, and lima beans have **15 grams per cup**.

White beans have the most protein with a whopping **17.42 grams per cup**.

Unlike animal sources of protein, **beans are virtually fat free**.

Fiber

Fiber is essential for many reasons. It helps to normalize bowel movements, maintain bowel health, lowers cholesterol levels, and helps to control blood sugar levels.

Beans are among the highest sources of dietary fiber, with the average cup of beans providing **14 grams of fiber**, which is **56% of the recommended daily intake**.

Iron

Iron is a component of red blood cells. If you aren't getting enough iron, it can lead to anemia as well as poor immune function. Iron deficiency is common in developing countries. Low-income American households also fall short of the necessary iron intake.

One-half cup of cooked red kidney beans provides **2.60 mg of iron**, which is **17% of the recommended daily**

intake of iron for men age 19 and older and **15% of the recommended daily value for women**.

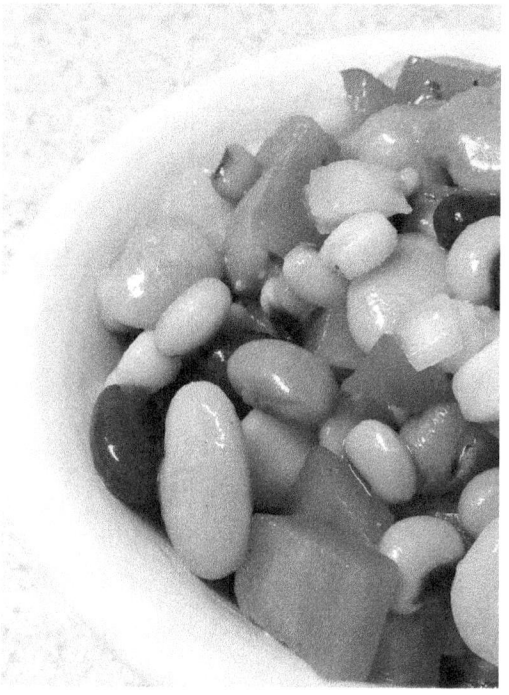

Folate

Folate is necessary for the formation of red blood cells. During pregnancy, folate is a key component for the development of the embryo, and inadequate intake can lead to serious birth defects.

One-half cup of cooked red kidney beans **provides 141mcg of folate**.

Antioxidants

Antioxidants are important substances that protect your cells against the effects of free radicals, which are produced in the body as it breaks down food and from exposure from pollutants.

Beans have the highest number of antioxidants among foods, even higher than cranberries and blueberries.

Magnesium

Magnesium is important for the production of energy as well as in the synthesis of the bones. There are more than three hundred metabolic reactions in the body that require magnesium.

One-half cup of navy beans contains 48mg of magnesium, which is over 10% of the recommended daily intake.

B Vitamins

There are eight B vitamins that all work together to keep our bodies running the way they are meant to.

The eight vitamins work both in tandem to help convert food into fuel, and to keep our bodies energized throughout the day. Various **beans are high in different B vitamins**.

Copper

Copper works with iron to help the body in the formation of red blood cells. Copper aids in the absorption of iron and helps to keep blood vessels, nerves, bones and the immune system healthy. **Kidney beans and white beans both contain 26% of the recommended daily intake of copper.**

Zinc

Zinc is responsible for our sense of smell and our sense of taste. It is also needed for the body's immune system to work properly. Zinc also plays a role in the division of cells, cell growth, wound healing, and aids in the breakdown of carbohydrates. **One cup of cooked baked beans contains 39% of the recommended daily value of zinc.**

Potassium

Potassium is needed to help regulate the balance of fluid in the body. It is important to maintain healthy blood pressure levels and is linked to improved bone health.

One-half cup of lima beans delivers 478mg of potassium, which is ten percent of the recommended daily intake.

Summary

It is clear to see that beans are an incredible source of many nutrients that are essential to our diets.

Being so high in so many nutrients and containing zero fat, beans are a great choice to add to your diet for many different reasons.

Health Benefits of Beans

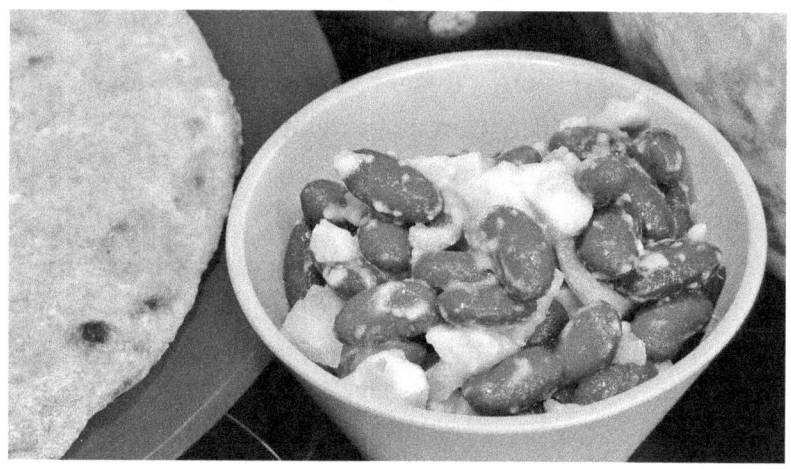

Being so high in so many nutrients, it comes as no surprise that beans also provide many different health benefits including heart health, lower cholesterol, optimal nutrition and healthy digestion.

Regulate Blood Sugar: Since beans are high in soluble fiber, they are excellent for limiting the spikes in glucose levels that occur after meals. If you suffer from insulin resistance, diabetes, or hypoglycemia adding beans into your regular diet is an effective way to help stabilize your blood sugar levels.

Lower Cholesterol: Beans contain no cholesterol and have been shown to be effective at lowering your cholesterol levels as well. Two separate research studies have shown that if you suffer from high cholesterol, eating one-half of a cup of beans each day for two months is enough to lower your cholesterol by twenty points.

If you pair beans with other foods that aid in lowering cholesterol, you can lower the points as effectively as you would statins.

Heart Health: Research that was done by the Department of Nutrition at the Harvard Medical School of Public Health found that eating just one serving of beans daily was found to yield a 38% decrease in the risk of myocardial infarction.

Beans contain no total cholesterol or LDL-cholesterol, both of which are directly correlated with heart disease. When the levels of cholesterol are lower, so is the risk of heart disease.

Digestive health: foods that are high in fiber, such as beans, are known to be beneficial to the health of our digestive tract. 20% of people over the age of sixty-five report suffering from constipation. Constipation is a condition that is often easily relieved by the consumption of foods that are high in fiber and low in fats, such as beans.

Weight Management and Weight Loss: A study that was done by the University of Washington School of Medicine showed that when people who put on a high protein diet they consumed 400 fewer calories per day than those who were consuming a lower protein diet.

The people in this study weren't given any limit to the amount of food they were allowed to consume, which shows us that when we consume a diet that is high in fiber, we feel full faster and longer than when we consume a less fiber rich diet.

Since beans are high in fiber and low in fat, they are an excellent choice if you are trying to lose weight, as well as for maintaining a healthy weight.

But What About Meat?

With beans being such a versatile food with so many benefits, it's a wonder they aren't consumed more frequently. Instead, many people opt to eat meat as their main source of protein. However, it does lead one to wonder if meat is the better option, or if we should replace some of our meat intake with beans.

Beans Versus Meat

Beans have been around for a long time and provide a very well packaged protein with the addition of many other nutritional benefits. They are typically well-liked by those who eat meat since they have a meaty taste, but how do they compare to meat proteins?

There are many different types of beans and meats. However, all of the beans were shown to have a very similar composition nutritionally. All beans contain the nine essential amino acids.

Meats, on the other hand, are not all created equal. For the purpose of this, we are going to compare canned dark red kidney beans to chicken, beef, and pork.

100 Gram Serving	Calories	Fat	Carbs	Protein	Fiber
Red Kidney Beans	127	0.5 grams; >1 gram saturated fat	22.8 grams	8.7 grams	6.4 grams
Grilled Chicken Breast	165	4 grams; 1 grams saturated fat	0	31 grams	0
80% Lean Ground Beef	272	17 grams; 7 grams saturated fat	0	27 grams	0
Grilled Top Loin Pork Chop	190	7 grams; 2 grams saturated fat	0	33 grams	0

Macronutrient Comparisons

Fiber

We already know that beans are high in soluble fiber, which makes them more filling than the meats. With obesity becoming such an epidemic, being able to consume a significantly smaller number of calories from beans over meats, makes beans the winner when it comes to caloric intake.

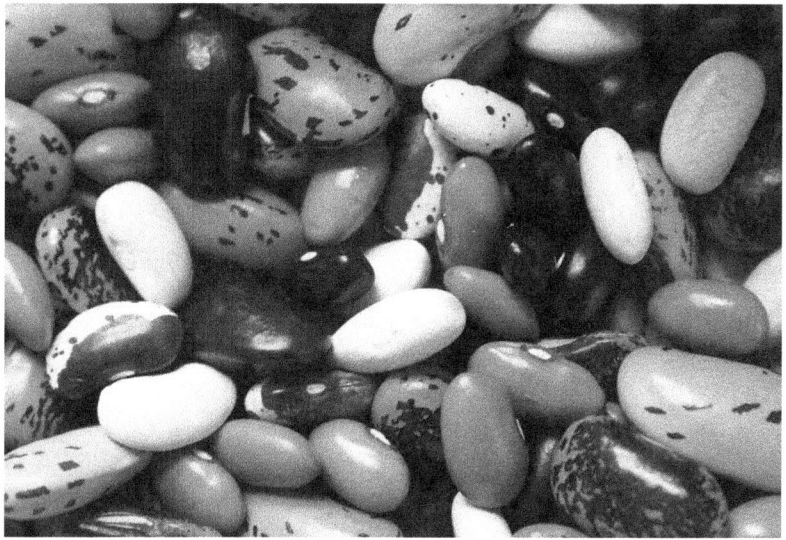

Carbs

Carbohydrates have been given a bad reputation, although they are an important part of a healthy diet, as long as they are consumed in a healthy form, known as complex carbs.

Carbohydrates are important for giving you both mental and physical energy. Neither chicken, beef or pork contain any carbohydrates. Again making beans the winner in this category.

Fat

When it comes to fat content, some fat is a good thing, but we know we don't want to overdo it. We know that monounsaturated fats are better for us than saturated fats. The meats that we compared above are all higher in saturated fats, while the beans are so low in fats, and the fats they do contain are monounsaturated fats, also known as the good fats.

Due to the extreme differences in the fat levels, beans are the clear winner.

Protein

The protein level in beans as compared to meat is pretty significant. If the only consideration to determine a winner was protein, the win would go to meat. However, this only really gives the meat a slight boost over beans. Beans contain enough protein that it is still reasonable for us to get the remainder of our protein from other sources.

The Cost Factor

Another aspect to beans that make them a better option than meat is cost. The USDA reports that one pound of beans costs just $1.07 while one pound of beef is around $5.28. There are also studies that back the opinion that beans are the better option over meats.

Beans Make a Great Meat Substitute

The Canadian Medical Association Journal showed that eating just half a cup of beans a day can reduce LDL, or bad, cholesterol, which a study that was published in Nutrients identified eating meats as a risk factor for developing diabetes.

One of the great thing about beans is that there are **many different varieties of beans** available to use in our diets, which make it easy to keep things interesting.

List of All Beans

There are many different types of beans and each one has similar benefits. Here we are going to list out all of the beans that you can add to your diet to reap all of the amazing benefits beans provide.

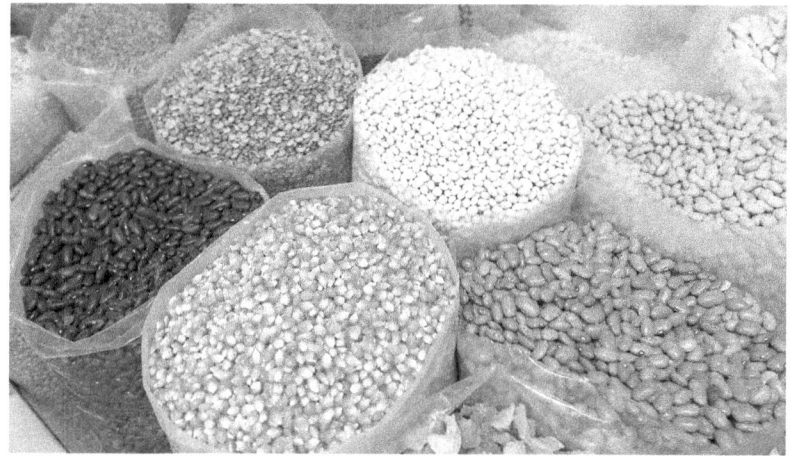

Azuki Beans – This is the bean that is used to make red bean paste. It is commonly used in Chinese and Japanese rice dishes.

Black Beans – Available in both dried and canned varieties. These beans have a velvety texture and a subtly sweet taste.

Black-Eyed Peas – These beans are small, plump, and spotted. They have an earthy flavor.

Butterbeans – This bean is similar to the popular Lima bean but smaller.

Cannellini Beans – Also known as White Italian Kidney Beans. These beans are creamy and have a delicate flavor.

Chinese Long Bean – This bean is slightly milder than a snap bean and has a crunchy texture. This bean is often used in stir-fries.

Cranberry Beans – These beans are used fresh or dried. They are common in stews and soups and have a flavor reminiscent of chestnuts.

Fava Bean – This bean can be eaten raw or cooked. They are added to soups and stews or used in salads.

Garbanzo Beans – Also known as chickpeas. These are the most consumed beans in the world. They are round and firm, have a nutty flavor and most known through Hummus.

Great Northern Beans – These beans are small, white, and shaped like kidneys. They have a mild flavor and easily absorb seasonings.

Green Beans – These beans are often sold fresh. They are sometimes called snap beans and are completely edible.

Kidney Beans – This bean is popular in chili and well known for its color and shape.

Lentil – this is a flat, disk-like seed that is used dry. While a lentil isn't specifically a bean, it is often lumped in with beans since it is similar in makeup and nutrients.

Lima Beans – These beans are often sold cooked and frozen. They are green, flat, and oval shaped. They have a buttery flavor and a starchy interior that can easily turn mushy.

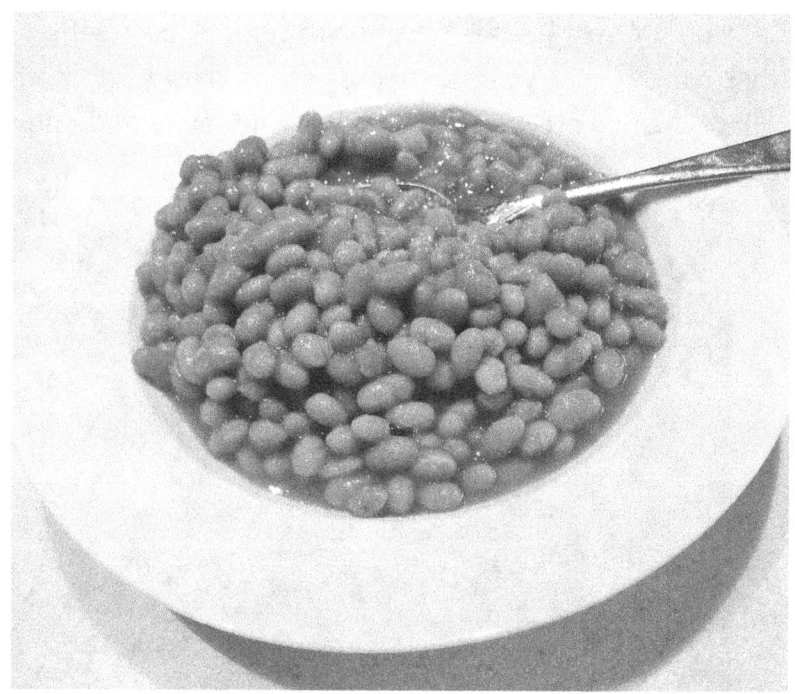

Mung Bean – This is a bean that is typically used to make bean meal. Used a lot in Indian, Chinese, and Asian cooking.

Navy Beans – This is a small, oval, kidney-shaped bean that is white in color. The name is thought to originate from its importance to the navy's shipboard kitchen stock.

Pinto Beans – This bean is light brown and has an earthy flavor. Its smooth texture works well in dips and stews.

Purple Snap Beans – These beans are a dried bean that turns from a dark purple color too green when cooked.

Scarlet Runner Beans – This bean is similar to the snap beans but contains more flavor. The bean is small and beige with red streaks and purple and black markings.

Soy Beans – These beans are tan to black with seeds that can be red, yellow, black, green, brown, or mottled. These beans are available dried and can be boiled in cooking.

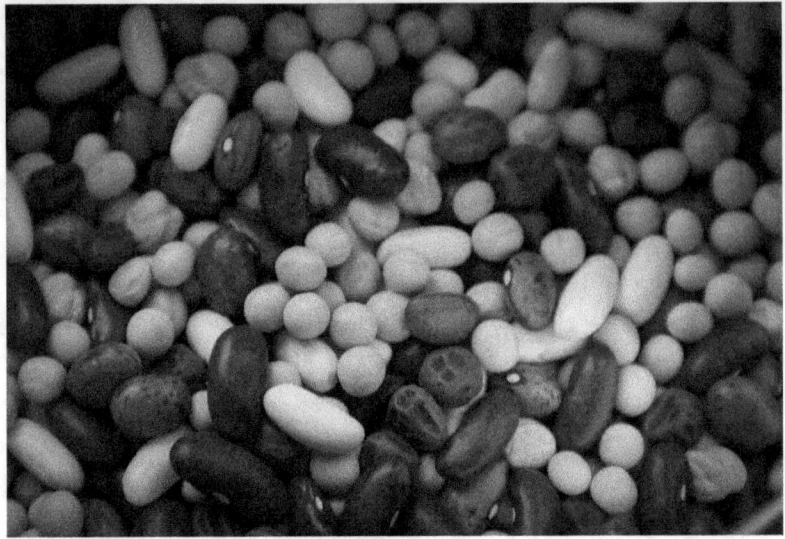

Wax Bean – This is a snap bean that is yellow in color and has a somewhat waxy texture, and delicious in salads.

Winged Beans – These beans are similar in flavor to the cranberry bean and can be steamed, roasted or dried to make them digestible.

There is no shortage of beans available for you to add into your diet. Each of these beans has a different flavor and texture making it easy to incorporate beans into your daily diet.

Eating and Cooking Ideas

Since we know that the goal is to incorporate beans into our daily eating habits, we are going to look at some options for where you can incorporate beans. We are going to look at breakfast, lunch, supper, and snacks.

Breakfast Options

Beans may not scream breakfast food to you, but there are numerous options for you to incorporate beans into your early morning meal.

The **appetite satisfaction and energy provided by beans make them a great choice for the first meal of the day.**

Breakfast Burrito – Make this similar to any other burrito you could make. To make it more breakfast friendly you can use a scrambled egg and vegetables that you would often put into an omelet. Add some black beans or refried beans.

Bean Chilaquiles – This is a breakfast dish that is made with tortillas, pinto beans, eggs, and salsa.

Baked Beans On Toast – This Breakfast is popular in Britain and can be served with a drizzle of malt vinegar. If you cook the beans until they are very soft and falling apart, the beans will be creamier and similar to peanut butter in texture.

Tofu Scramble – You can add some cooked beans to any tofu scramble, or egg scramble.

Ful Medammes – This is an Egyptian and Arabic breakfast that is made with fava beans, olive oil, garlic, and lemon juice. It is typically served with pita bread.

Lunch Options

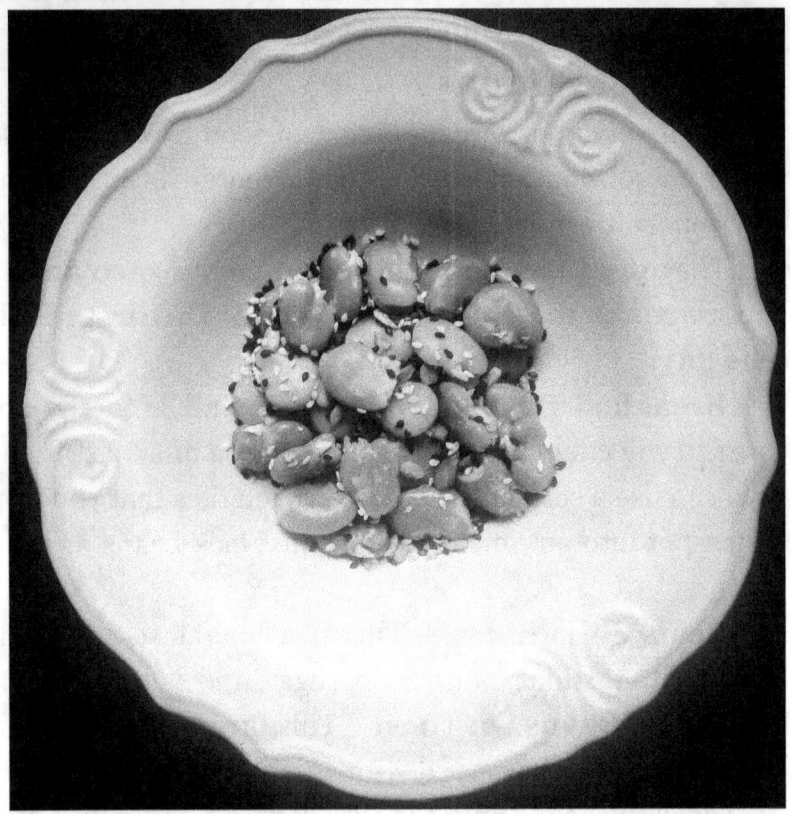

Having beans for lunch may make it seem as though you are going to be eating some bean salad every day with no real variety, but this is the far from the truth.

Middle Eastern Wrap – This wrap is made with garlic, cucumber, olives, red pepper, tomatoes, and any other vegetables you wish to add. You can use almost any of the kidney beans in this recipe, as you would like as you are going to puree the bean.

Bean Pasta – This can be made with any short pasta you choose to use. You can then add bell peppers, tomatoes, olives, and parmesan cheese. Northern white beans go great with this recipe.

Bean Soup – This soup is going to be similar to a vegetable soup, with the addition of any beans of your choosing.

Bean and Cheese Dip – This dip is super easy to make. Mash up some beans and top them with some grated parmesan cheese. Throw it into the microwave for a few seconds and use it as a dip for pita bread and vegetables of your choosing.

Supper Options

When you think of bean recipes, you probably instantly think of a chili. In our supper ideas, we are going to show you some ideas that are a little different from the typical chilies and enchiladas you usually think of.

Savory Stuffed Sweet Potatoes with White Beans and Kale – This is an easy meal that only requires sweet potatoes, kale, some seasonings, and cooked and drained white beans. Since it is cooked in the oven, it doesn't require you to be very hands-on to make, which makes it perfect when you are multitasking.

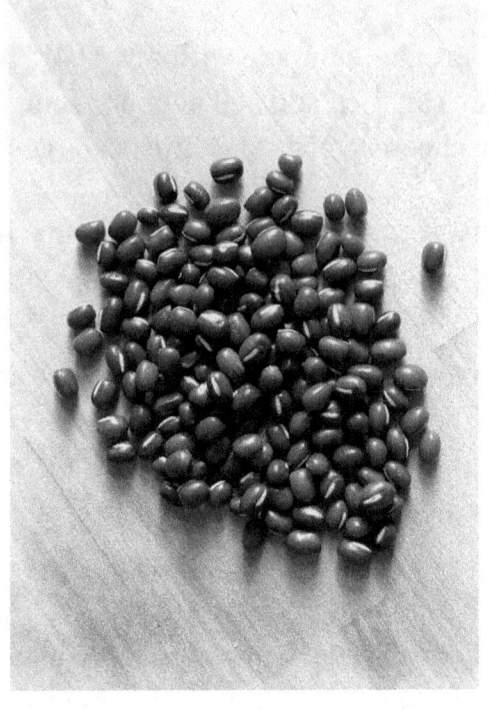

Southwestern Pizza with Black Beans and Corn – Everyone loves pizza, and this will be no exception. Made with pizza dough, frozen corn, cheese, some seasonings and one can of drained and rinsed black beans, you will be enjoying a delicious pizza in no time.

Summer Squash and White Bean Sauté – This sauté is extremely versatile and works with eggplant, peppers, or corn. You can serve it with rice of bulgur.

Beans in Tomato Sauce with Creamy Polenta – this recipe is simple and elegant and will warm you up from the inside on a cold winter's day.

Snack Options

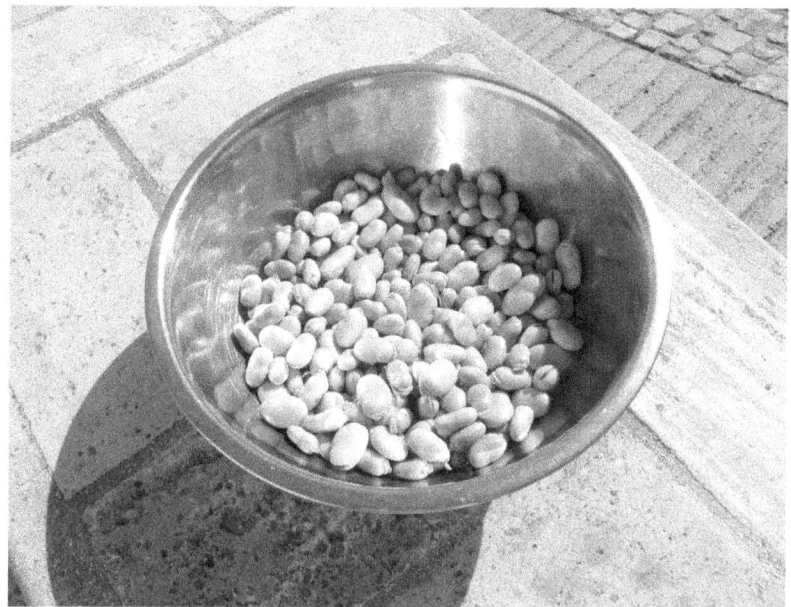

When it comes to snack foods, beans probably don't make your list as all. Here are some great options to bring beans into your snacking routine, without feeling awkward or being limited to hummus.

Roasted Beans – To make roasted beans, all you have to do is sprinkle some garbanzo beans with some olive oil and cook them in the oven for half of an hour at 400 degrees. These roasted beans can be eaten on their own, or used in a trail mix.

Crispy Green Bean Chips – This is an easy recipe to make, it only calls for beans, oil, salt and garlic and onion powders. Mix everything together and place in a dehydrator or an oven at a low temperature until they are crispy.

Hummus – Hummus is a wonderful choice made from pureed chickpeas and comes in many flavors to make a healthy, low fat and nutrient rich snack for dipping vegetables or whole grain crackers.

Cooking Beans

For many people, dried beans seem a little scary and overwhelming, however, they are not overly complicated to cook.

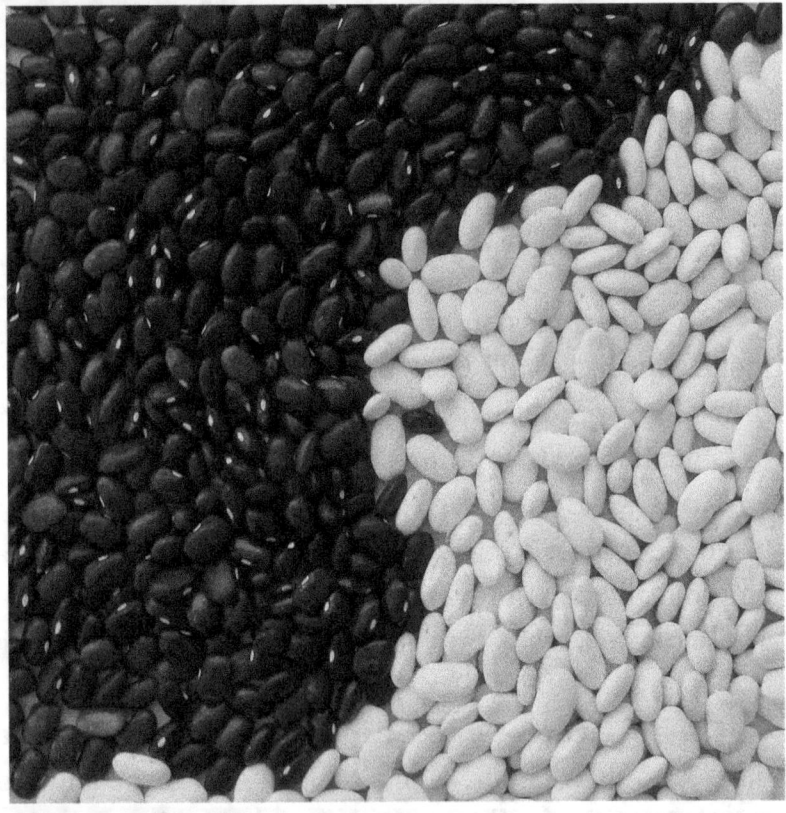

Soaking Beans

First, it is important to know that you are going to get better results if you soak your dried beans before you are going to be cooking them. This isn't necessary, but it will speed up the cooking process.

To properly soak beans, place them in a large container and add water so it is about 2 inches over the top of the beans. You are going to want to leave them overnight, or for at least eight hours before you drain them and get ready to cook them.

Cooking Methods

On The Stove – It is important to know that good beans take a long time. You are going to want to cover your beans with at least one inch of water before you place them on the stove.

Bring to a boil over a medium-high heat and then reduce to a simmer for the rest of the cooking time. You should barely see the water boil; this will ensure the beans are cooked evenly and won't turn to mush.

Beans can also be simmered in other liquids, like chicken broth, which all add loads of flavor.

In The Oven – This is less conventional but incredibly easy. Preheat your oven to 325F. Place the beans into an ovenproof pot such as a Dutch oven and cover them with one inch of water. Bring the beans to a boil on the stove and then place them in the over until they are done, about 75 minutes.

In The Slow Cooker – Place your beans in the slow cooker and cover with at least one inch of water. Cook on low for six to eight hours. Start checking them after the five-hour mark.

Additionally, many complete meals can be made in the slow cooker by adding various vegetables, and liquids to the beans, for example onions, garlic, and tomatoes. Many recipes are available online, and using a slow cooker will allow you to have a virtually effort free, ready-made, hot and highly nutritious bean meal when you get home from work.

In The Pressure Cooker – This is by far the fastest method and can make edible beans in less than an hour. To use this method, you need to presoak your beans. Place your drained beans into the pressure cooker, and add your aromatics and eight cups of water.

Cook according to your model of pressure cooker's instruction manual, allowing the pot to reach high pressure before you reduce it too medium and begin timing. Allow the pot too cool and release the pressure on its own.

Final Thoughts on Beans

Not only are beans a healthy alternative to meats for virtually fat free protein, they also provide you with complex carbs for energy, fiber, iron, and so many other vitamins and minerals. They also cost much less than meat, and give you a healthy choice for weight loss and weight management.

Beans are never boring, and offer many different cooking and eating options. The ample variety in types of beans each with their own distinct flavors is reason enough to add them to your weekly menus to make for diverse and tasty meals.

If you are looking for a simple way to add more plant-based proteins into your diet, beans are the way to go!

Tofu Guide

What Is Tofu

Tofu is a soy-based food product that originated in China and is made in a very similar way to cheese. There is a story that tofu was first created by accident over two thousand years ago when a Chinese chef accidentally dropped soymilk into some nigari.

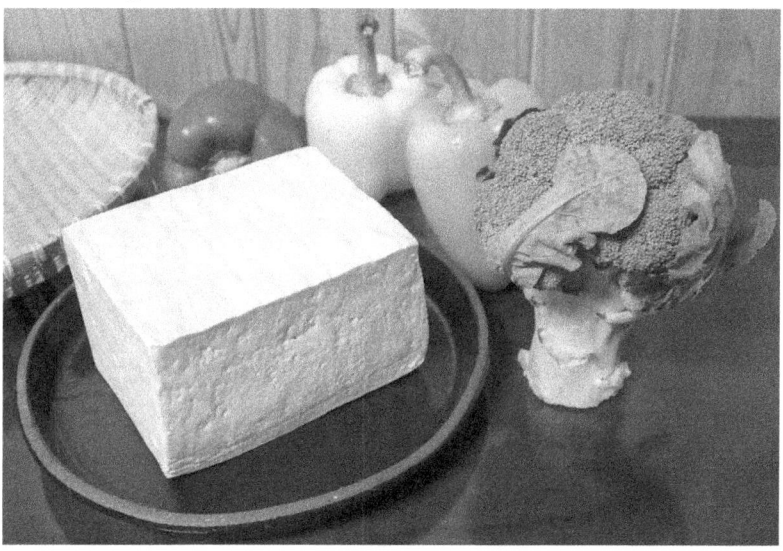

Nigari is a mineral-rich coagulant that is used to curdle tofu by making it condense and hold its shape when it is pressed into blocks. Tofu is also known by the name soya curd.

Tofu by itself is quite bland and lacks its own flavor; however, it readily absorbs the flavors of any other foods it is cooked with, including liquids.

Tofu is usually sold packaged in fluid and should be kept in this fluid and refrigerated until it is all used. Tofu can also be stored in the freezer or up to three months, but this will change its texture and make it much chewier.

Since tofu is known for being able to absorb the flavor of whatever it is cooked in, making it a very versatile animal protein substitute and delicious in many different recipes, both sweet and savory.

Three Types of Tofu

There are three commonly sold types of tofu, firm, soft, and silken.

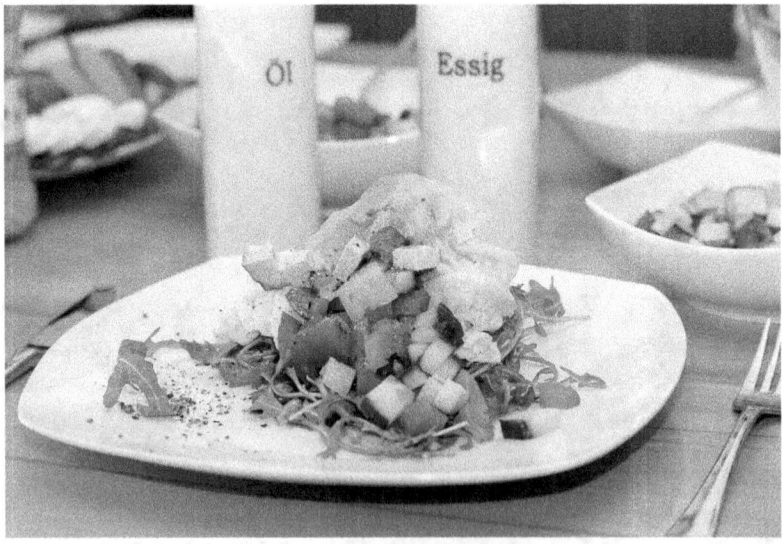

Firm Tofu

Firm tofu is very dense and can easily be cut into cubes or strips and then fried, baked, grilled, or served in soups. Firm tofu contains more protein and calcium than other types of tofu.

Soft Tofu

Soft tofu is usually used when a recipe requires for tofu to be blended or mashed. Silken tofu is common in Japanese cuisine and is much creamier than firm or soft tofu.

Silken Tofu

Silken tofu can also be used in place of egg in many recipes such as cheesecakes and pies.

Nutrients in Tofu

Soy has been recognized in Asia for thousands of years as a food high in nutritional value and as an excellent source of protein. In the modern West, respected nutritionists, dieticians, and doctors agree.

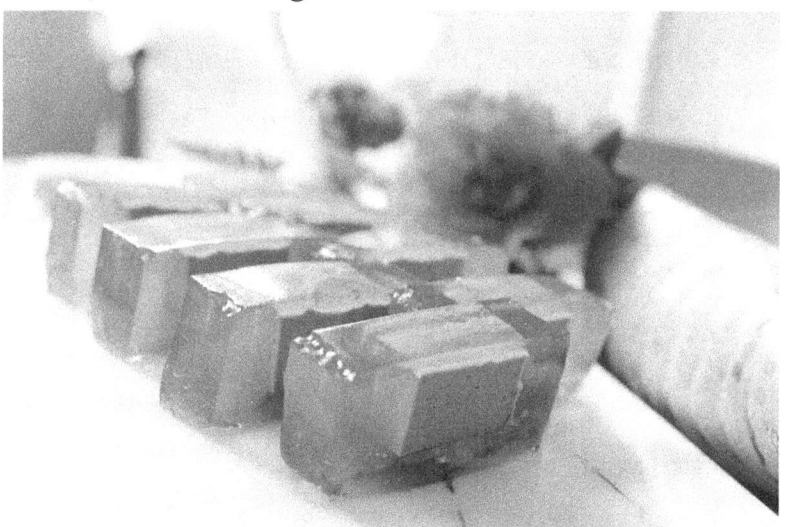

The soybean is amazing in that it contains all nine essential amino acids: histidine, isoleucine, leucine, lysine, methionine, phenylalanine, threonine, tryptophan, and valine.

The soybean also contains a number of other vitamins and minerals, including iron, calcium, magnesium, manganese, phosphorus, potassium, B group vitamins, zinc and vitamin C.

Soy also contains omega-3 and omega-6 fatty acids, and as high in fiber.

Depending on how the soybean is prepared, the concentrations of these nutrients and minerals vary, but are present in very high quantities in tofu.

A 100-Gram Serving of Tofu Contains:

- ✓ 31% of your Recommended Daily Intake (RDI) of manganese
- ✓ 20% of your RDI of calcium
- ✓ 14% of your RDI of selenium
- ✓ 12% of your RDI of phosphorus
- ✓ 9% of your RDI of magnesium
- ✓ 9% of your RDI of iron
- ✓ 6% of your RDI of zinc
- ✓ 11% of your RDI of copper

That is a huge number of minerals to be served in a tiny 100-gram portion of food.

This serving size also contains only 70 calories, making it a food very dense in nutrients.

Calories: Tofu Versus Animal Protein

Tofu is much lower in calories than equivalent servings of animal protein.

Tofu Versus Beef

A 250-gram, cup-sized, serving of tofu **has only 175 calories.**

The same portion of beef contains 625 calories, that's a massive 3.3x more calories in the same serving.

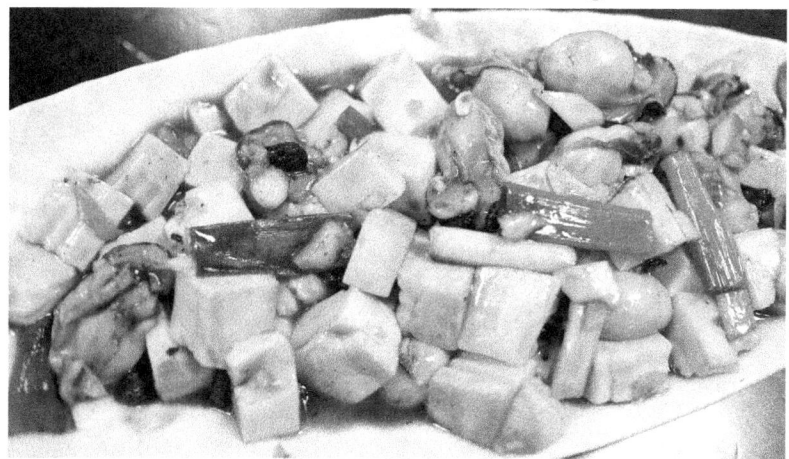

White Meat Versus Tofu

White meats, though often seen as a light or healthy choice compared to red meat, are also much higher in calories.

A 250-gram serving of chicken contains 598 calories, and a serving of the same size of salmon contains 520 calories.

Tofu is therefore a much better choice than animal protein for those looking to lose weight,

consume fewer calories, and yet maintain an optimal level of protein intake.

The Health Benefits of Tofu

Fiber

A cup of tofu contains 2.25 grams of fiber while red meat, chicken, and fish have no fiber.

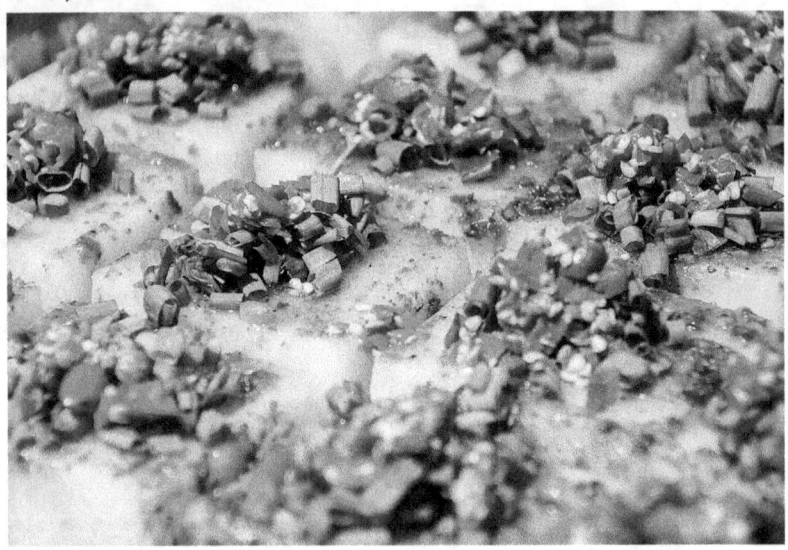

The fiber within tofu is extremely good for your body in many different ways. A high fiber diet can normalize your bowel movements, maintain bowel health, lower your cholesterol levels, control your blood sugar levels, and help you to stay at a healthy weight.

Consuming dietary fiber creates stools that are larger, heavier and softer, making them easier to pass, and lowering your risk of having constipation.

In contrast, meat products have been shown to cause constipation. Healthy bowel function is incredibly important because it decreases your chances of developing diseases in your colon, such as bowel cancer.

The soluble fiber found in tofu helps to decrease your overall blood cholesterol levels. It does this by lowering the "bad" cholesterol levels, low-density lipoprotein.

Studies also indicate that high-fiber foods can also reduce blood pressure and inflammation in the body.

The soluble fiber in tofu can also improve your blood sugar levels and slow down the rate at which sugar is absorbed into your body. This lowers your risk of developing type 2 diabetes.

Reduces Risks for Heart Disease

Tofu, unlike red meat and even white meat is not plagued with saturated fat, which is a known culprit in increasing risk factors for heart disease, and high cholesterol.

While animal protein certainly has its own set of nutritional and health benefits, it is wise to replace it in some meals with tofu to reduce your intake of saturated fat.

Supports Healthy Weight Management

Because tofu is full of nutrients, fiber and protein, but low in calories, it can **assist with weight** loss by **decreasing your overall caloric consumption and keeping you feeling fuller for longer.** Reducing your weight to a healthy Body Mass Index (BMI) level is incredibly important to keeping your body healthy.

Obesity is linked to a number of diseases such as heart disease, fatal cardiovascular disease, stroke, high blood pressure, type 2 diabetes, gout, osteoarthritis, gallbladder disease, gallstones, asthma, and sleep apnea. Obesity is also linked to cancers of the breast, uterus, colon, and rectum.

Reduce Risks for Cancer

Swapping meat for tofu can also reduce your risk of breast and prostate cancers.

This is due to the major isoflavone in soy, genistein, which contains antioxidant properties. Genistein inhibits the growth of cancer cells. A study published in the medical journal Environmental Health Perspectives has shown that consuming at least 10 milligrams of soy per day can actually decrease the recurrence of breast cancer by 25%.

Sufferers of type 2 diabetes often develop kidney disease, which causes their bodies to excrete high amounts of protein in their urine. A recent study from the University of Illinois found that people, who only consumed soy protein in their diet, and not meat, excreted less protein in their urine.

The isoflavones found in soy are known to increase bone mineral density and to prevent bone loss during menopause. They have also been found to reduce other menopausal symptoms, so tofu may produce many noticeable health benefits for women experiencing menopause.

Prevent Liver Damage

Studies from Ibrahim Badamasi Babangida University and the Federal University of Technology in Nigeria have shown that tofu, in all of its types owing to its own natural properties and its curdling with a coagulant, can actually prevent liver damage caused by free radicals.

Possibly Reduce Risks for Dementia

Age-related brain diseases such as dementia and Alzheimer's disease could also be prevented by soy consumption. Based on epidemiological findings, analyzed geographically, it has been observed by researchers at the National Institute of Environmental Health Sciences that populations that consume high amounts of soy generally have lower levels of age-related brain diseases.

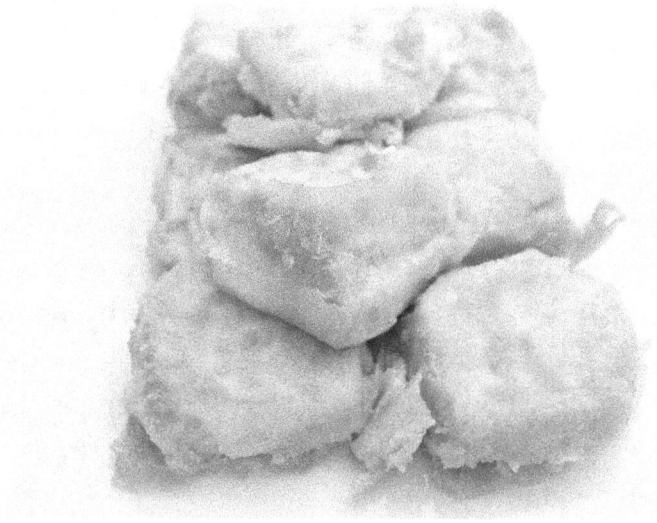

Nutrition: Soy Protein Versus Animal Protein

Animal meat contains higher levels of protein per gram than soy. To gain the same amount of protein as beef, you would have to consume 3.25 times more tofu.

However, tofu contains far more nutrients, essential acids, and minerals while being lower in calories.

100 grams of beef will provide you with 26 grams of protein, but contains 250 calories, only 1% of the RDI of calcium and 15 grams of fat.

You can get the same 26 grams of protein from 325 grams of tofu, with 227.5 calories, more than RDI of calcium (113.75%) and 15 grams of fat also.

This makes soy overall, the healthier choice over animal protein as it is lower in calories and provides more vitamins and minerals. Consuming a larger volume of food will also keep you feeling fuller for longer.

Soy protein, that tofu is made from, lowers levels of bad cholesterol, and contains phytoestrogens called isoflavones - a set of natural chemicals found in some plants, and soy foods.

They are structured similarly to the female human hormone estrogen and they act similarly to estrogen produced by the body. They bind naturally to estrogen receptor sites in a range of human cells including breast tissue cells, and this is shown to actually reduce the risks of some cancers including breast cancer.

GMO Tofu Versus Organic Non-GMO Tofu

There is a lot of controversy around foods that are grown from genetically modified organism (GMO) crops. GMO crops are very new in the grand scheme of human agricultural cultivation, which began approximately 10,000 years ago.

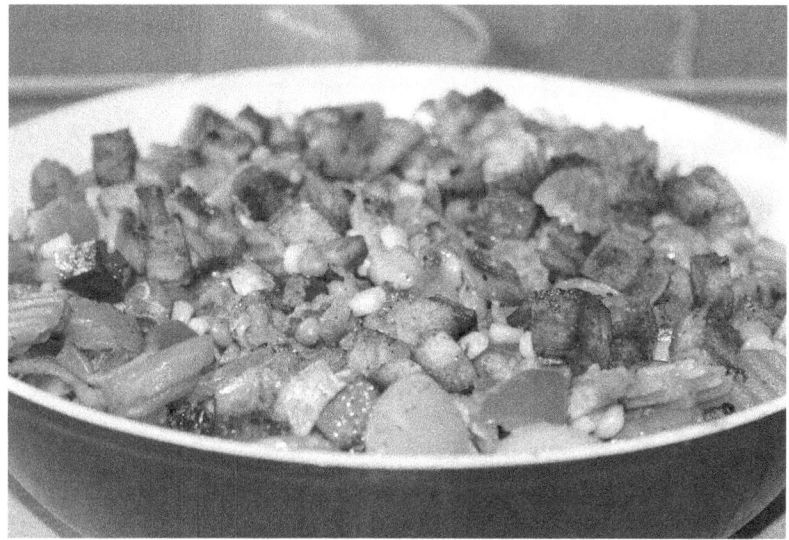

Many of the new GMO crops that exist in the world have not existed long enough to be studied rigorously and we simply **do not know the long-term effects of these GMO products on our health**. For this reason, many people avoid GMO products in favor of organic, non-GMO foods.

It is important to note that the largest consumer of commercially grown GMO soy products, both in the United States and internationally, is actually livestock.

By consuming meat products, you are actually consuming the byproducts of ingested GMO soy and the affects that these have had on the animal's biological makeup.

It is estimated that **80% of all soybean crops globally are GMO, and 85% of those GMO crops end up as feed for livestock**. When dairy animals or livestock for slaughter consume GMO soy protein, those proteins end up being passed on to you when you consume those animal products.

Many **organic, non-GMO tofu products are available to buy in supermarkets** and if you are concerned about the implications of GMO products on your health, this may be the choice you wish to make.

In Europe, the United States, and Australia, these products will very clearly be labeled non-GMO.

The Versatility of Eating and Cooking with Tofu

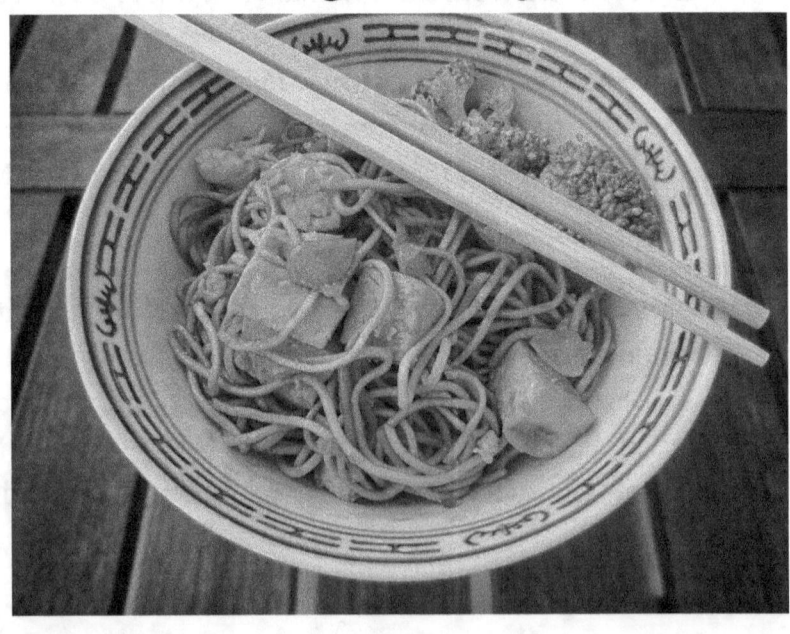

You can find tofu in large, bulk packages, or smaller individual packages. The tofu will always be suspended in water when sold to you, often in a sealed container or a vacuum package that is sold at room temperature.

Storing Tofu

You need to keep your tofu refrigerated once these packs have been opened. Once the tofu is opened, you should rinse it, cover it with water and keep it in a sealed container (in the refrigerator, remember!).

Continue to rinse the tofu and change the water it is kept in while it stays in your fridge daily, in order to keep it fresh.

You should consume all tofu within a week, otherwise bacterial or fungal growth may be present with risks of food poisoning, so use caution just like you would with meat products.

You can also freeze the tofu for up to three months, but the tofu will change in consistency becoming much tougher and chewier when you defrost it. It should be defrosted at room temperature, avoid doing this in a microwave.

Tofu Options

You can buy tofu that has already been marinated at the supermarket. This is a great option for newcomers to tofu, as it has no real taste or flavor of its own. You may feel adventurous and try to buy and cook a package of firm tofu, only to find that it tastes terrible and then all of your enthusiasm will be lost.

If you are unfamiliar with the preparation of tofu, you may want to stick to these pre-flavored options and then move onto other recipes once you gain more confidence.

As firm, soft and silken tofu varieties all have very different consistencies and tofu itself essentially has no taste, it is incredibly versatile. You can use tofu as a meat or egg substitute in basically any food, or in any type of international cuisine.

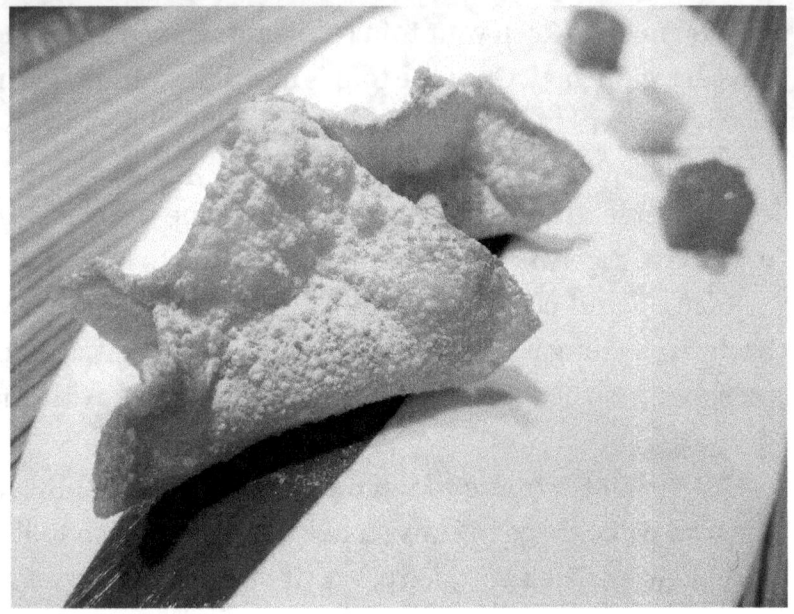

Soft and Silken Tofu Can Be Used in:

- Sauces
- Shakes
- Salad dressings
- Desserts
- Puddings, you name it!

Firm Tofu Can Be:

- Cut into shapes and grilled
- Stir-fried
- Baked
- Any other way you would cook a meat product

The Possibilities Are Unlimited!

You can make burgers, sausages, kebab skewers and all kinds of other barbecue foods out of tofu.

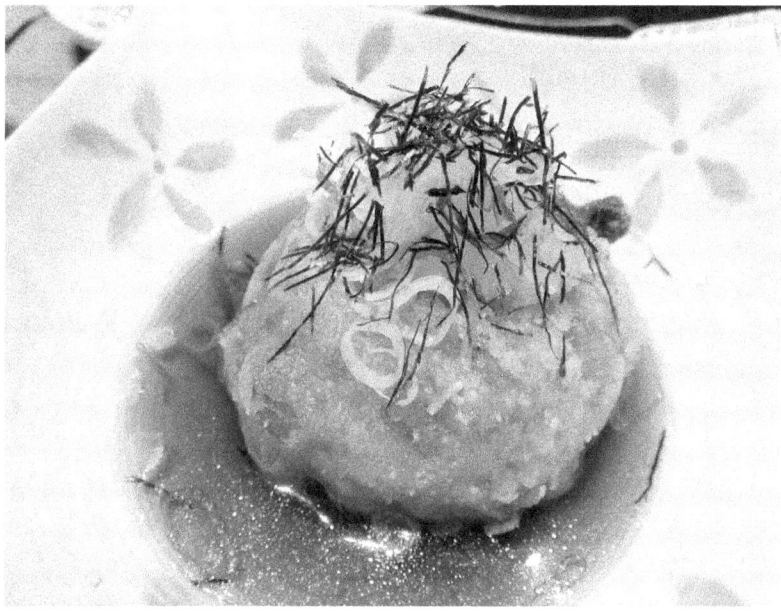

You could fry finely chopped tofu with garlic and onion and adding it to your pasta sauces or salads, cutting it up into strips and adding it to your curry, or adding silken tofu to your fruit smoothie for extra protein.

The only limits of tofu are your imagination!

Tofu Recipes

Here are three excellent recipes that you could try:

1. Blueberry Banana Tofu Smoothie

Ingredients:

- 2 cups fresh blueberries
- 1 large banana
- 3 tbsp. honey
- 3/4 cup milk
- 6 oz. silken tofu
- 1/2 cup ice

Method:

Add all ingredients to a blender and mix well. Pour into a glass and enjoy. Too easy!

2. Vegetarian Thai Red Curry Soup

Ingredients:

- 1 Tbs. coconut oil
- 12 oz. firm tofu, cubed
- 4 large green onions, thinly sliced and green and white parts cut and separated
- 2 Tbs. Thai red curry paste
- 4 cups low-sodium vegetable broth

- 1 15-oz. can diced tomatoes
- 3/4 cup light coconut milk
- 6 oz. green beans, cut into 1-inch pieces
- 1 Tbs. lime juice

Method:

1. Heat coconut oil in a large saucepan over medium heat.
2. Add the diced tofu and white parts of green onions. Sauté these for about four minutes, or until they begin to brown.
3. Stir in curry paste, and sauté for one more minute.
4. Add the vegetable broth and tomatoes.
5. Bring to a boil, and then reduce the heat to a simmer with a medium-low heat.
6. Simmer for five minutes.
7. Add coconut milk and green beans.
8. Simmer for another ten minutes.
9. Remove from heat. Serve in a bowl with lime juice and remaining green onions stirred in.

3. Dairy-Free Tofu Cheesecake

Ingredients:

- 2 cups of graham cracker crumbs
- 1/4 cup organic maple syrup
- 1/4 tsp. almond extract
- 1 lb. firm silken tofu
- 1/3 cup brown sugar
- 1 Tbs. almond butter
- 1/2 tsp. salt
- 1 to 2 tsp. grated orange rind
- 1 Tbs. cornstarch dissolved in 2 Tbs. soy milk
- 1 Tbs. coconut oil

Method:
Crust:
Preheat oven to 350 degrees (F).

1. Mix graham cracker crumbs, organic maple syrup, and almond extract in a large bowl until the crumbs are completely moistened.
2. Use coconut oil to grease a 9-inch pie dish.
3. Pour the crumb mixture into the dish.
4. Press the mixture firmly to form a crust.
5. Bake for just 5 minutes, then remove from the oven and let the crust cool while preparing the filling.

Filling:

In a blender, combine remaining ingredients and blend on medium speed until smooth, which should take about 30 seconds.

Pour the filling mixture into the cooled crust.

Bake until top is slightly browned. This should take around about 30 minutes.

Refrigerate the cake for around two hours until thoroughly chilled and firm. Serve and enjoy!

Precautions

Tofu is considered to be generally safe for consumption, though some considerations apply and intake may have to be moderated under these conditions, (ask your doctor):

- ✓ If you have kidney or gallbladder stones, tofu may worsen these conditions because it contain oxalates, though not all researchers agree, and some actually believe soy can improve kidney stones, ask your doctor.
- ✓ If you have breast tumors, doctors recommend limiting soy intake. Again, as your doctor, as research from the European Food Safety Authority (EFSA) found that soy isoflavones pose no threat to breast or uterine cancers.
- ✓ Doctors also advise those with thyroid issues to avoid tofu due to its nitrogen content.

- ✓ Infants should not be exposed to soy isoflavones as they can disrupt the development of reproductive organs.
- ✓ While no human studies exist, animal studies suggest that ingesting high amounts of soy may interfere with fertility.

Other Meat Alternatives

You have other choices when it comes to meat and animal protein alternatives, which are 100% vegan.

Tempeh

Tempeh is made by fermenting cooked soybeans with a mold. It comes in flat rectangular shapes, which are approximately 8 inches long. Tempeh is a brownish color and has a firm and chewy texture with a hearty sweet flavor.

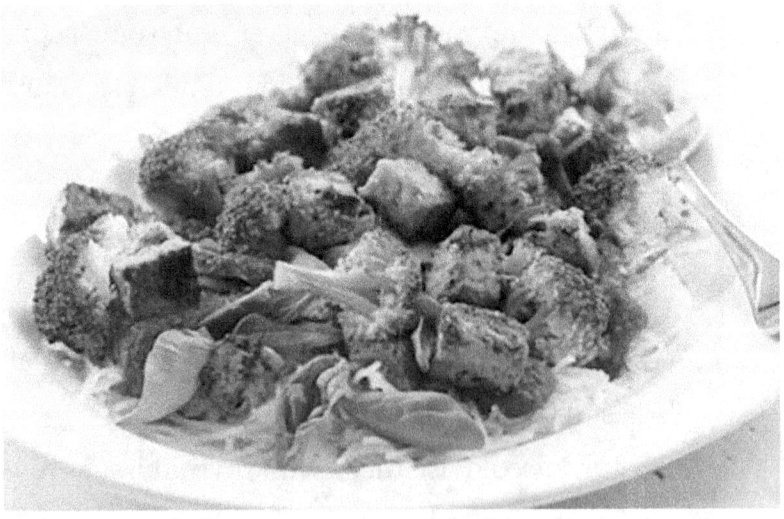

Tempeh as compared to tofu has more calories and less fiber but more protein. It is also **less processed than tofu**.

Tempeh is **much chewier than tofu** and is **less versatile when used in recipes** as tofu offers various textures that can be easier manipulated in savory and sweet dishes.

Nevertheless, **tempeh can be marinated, seasoned, steamed, grilled, blackened, and baked.**

It goes great with various vegetables and grains and in both hot and cold dishes like salads. It can also be crumbled for use in stews and sauces.

Like tofu, it **does a great job of taking on the flavor of whatever it is cooked** in making it a versatile animal protein substitute in your favorite meal.

Many recipes use Tempeh, including, stews, curries, chilies, and pasta sauces.

Meat Analogs

There are various soy meat alternatives, sometimes referred to as "meat analogs," which are made from soy proteins and wheat gluten. Some are also made with tofu and ready to eat from the package. These foods are convenient, and are usually flavored, and seasoned and ready to eat.

These products are vegan and vegetarian, and they very much resemble your favorite meat products, like bacon, sausage, burgers, and the like so they make great substitutes for animal protein.

Meat Alternatives Include

- Sausage links and crumbles
- Bacon
- Sausage patties and links
- Soy burgers
- Chicken patties and nuggets
- Hot Dogs
- Stews
- Chili
- Taco filling
- Veggie burgers
- And many others

Suppliers and Brands

- ✓ Boca Foods/Kraft™
- ✓ MorningStar Farms™
- ✓ Hain Celestial Group, Inc.™
- ✓ Pulmuone Wildwood™

Final Thoughts

Given the amazing number of health benefits from going meatless and consuming tofu, it seems like a very intelligent option to try it out.

The versatility of tofu makes a great very low fat high protein alternative to meat. One thing is sure, not only vegan and vegetarians can benefit from this unique soy meat alternative.

If you currently eat a lot of meat, you may want to start small by simply swapping one of your major meals per week from meat to tofu.

As you learn to cook with tofu, adjust to the taste, and reap the health benefits, you may want to go meatless more and more often.

Stay well and take care!

Dos and Don'ts of Vegetarian Diet

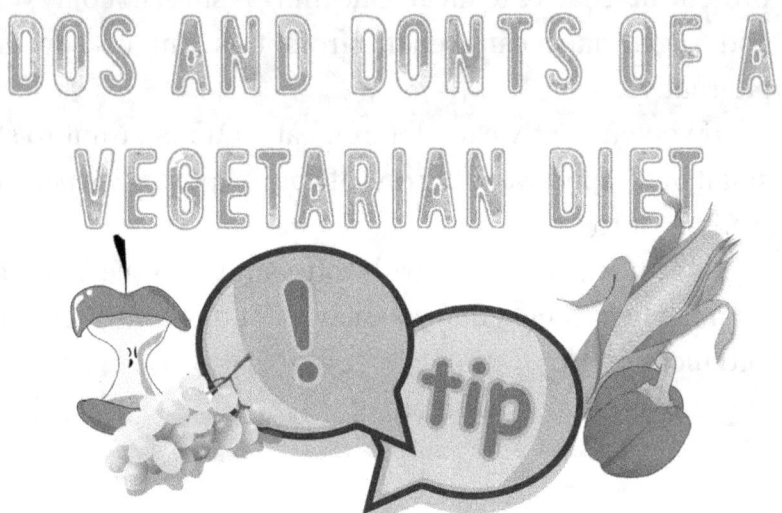

Vegetarianism is a healthy and life prolonging diet choice. According to a study by the National Institutes of Health, vegetarians had lower rates of death from things like cardiovascular disease, diabetes, and even kidney failure. These are great motivators to get started on a vegetarian diet, but before you do there are some do's and don'ts that you will want to follow to ensure that you have the best experience.

What You Should Do
Eat Whole Food and Avoid the Processed

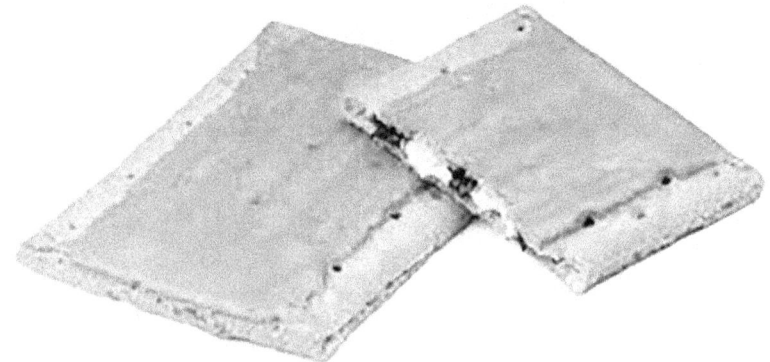

Fast fix and instant foods are a very tempting option when you're cruising through the frozen section of your grocery store. Unfortunately, the processes that these foods go through remove many of the natural nutrients and add things our bodies don't need. Avoiding processed foods will help ensure you get the most out of your vegetarian diet. Instead, make sure you're eating a wide variety of whole foods that are unprocessed and one ingredient. This gives you a huge variety of options from things like beans and nuts, to whole grains to fruits and vegetables, like avocados, zucchini, berries, and coconut.

Do Make Your Favorite Foods Just Make Them Vegetarian

As previously mentioned, most any of your favorite foods can be made without meat. Beans are a great swap when it comes to replacing meat in a regular dish, milk can be replaced with almond or soymilk and cheese with soy cheeses. You don't have to avoid the things you love you just have to re-think them and do the research to find appropriate vegetarian recipes and substitutes.

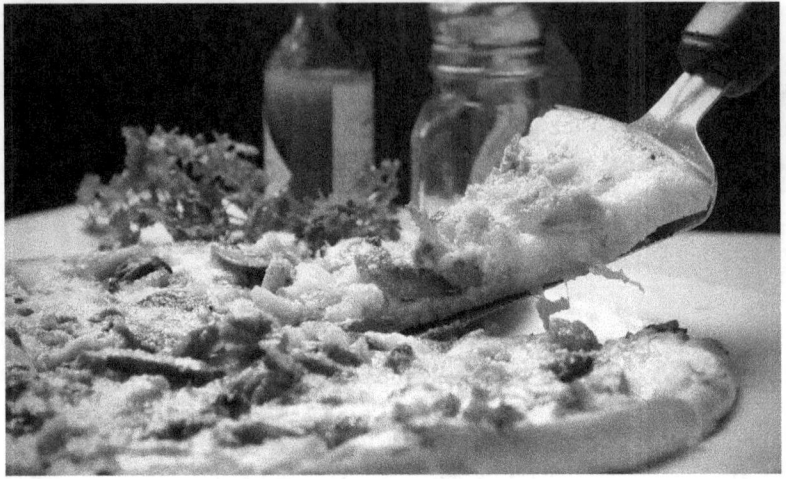

Do Consult with A Nutritionist

A nutritionist or dietician can be a great asset when first starting the journey to a meat free lifestyle. They can help establish a sound nutritional plan that includes the foods you like to eat, makes the whole process hands free and most medical plans cover this service.

Do Remember Why You Started

Quitting meat can be difficult, there will be times when you will crave a cheeseburger or steak, and it's at these times when it is really important to remember why you started a plant diet. It is useful to make a list of the reasons before you start that you can refer to as needed.

Do Get Support

It's always a good idea to have people in your life who are also vegetarian or vegan.

Do Get Excited

Get excited about your new lifestyle choice and support your family in getting excited! You are doing something good for your health.

What You Should Not Do

Don't Forget the Protein

Protein is an absolute necessity. Thankfully, you have lots of options and a good variety when it comes to choosing your protein. Many vegetarian and vegan friendly foods contain protein, and there are many great substitutions so you can enjoy burgers, tacos, and chili without the beef and stir fry and kabobs without the chicken.

Don't Be Afraid of Tofu, Tempeh and Other Soy Proteins

It can be intimidating to look at a package that contains a white cube, and not have any clue as to what to do with it. Do not let fear keep you from using these great soy products to replace meat in your recipes. Go online or buy a book on how to use them and begin to experiment with recipes, before you know it you will be an expert.

Don't Forget the Supplements

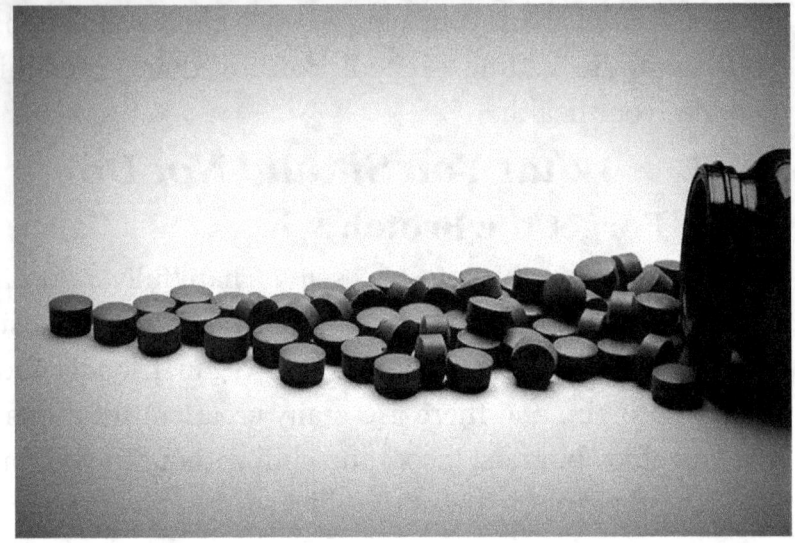

One of the biggest mistakes vegans and vegetarians can make is not addressing their supplement needs. Supplements can be incredibly important for having a healthy well-rounded diet when you are a vegetarian. The first on this list is B12. B12 is the superhero of vitamins; it supports nerve and blood cell function, is key to oxygen moving through the body, and helps your body make DNA. Because this vitamin is such a superhero it's not one you will want to do without, however the primary source for this wonder vitamin happens to be found in beef and liver.

This doesn't mean you have to do without because many foods are fortified with B12 and you can get it as a supplement. When you are picking a food or drink that has been supplemented make sure that the label reads at least 25%.

Daily vitamins are also a good way to ensure that you are getting a balanced and healthy amount of the nutrients you need in addition to your regular diet. Ask your doctor or nutritionist about supplements you may need.

About the Author

Rod is an author, publisher, consultant, and provider of information on health, nutrition and work from home in order to improve your life.

Rod is the principle partner of **Rod Stone Group** and the r Healthy Living Solutions, where they focus on providing information on health, nutrition, and work from home in order to improve your life. They also provide publishing assistance via book graphics and other assistance. With over two dozen experts providing content, they are able to provide some of the most useful information you will find.

Rod began writing articles on health and nutrition in the mid '90s. In 2004 he started full time working with people and providing information and products to assist with health and nutrition. In 2008 he started to become involved with the importance of specialized high intensity workouts.

The following are some books that relate well to this work that can all be found on Amazon

Nutrients for Health: your guide to foods and nutrients for your health and for overcoming ailments

Learning to Eat Healthy: find out what your body needs and how to shop; store; and prepare for the best in taste

Vegetables: Learn to Enjoy More Varieties While Benefitting Your Health

Vegetable recipes from the past: learn how to enjoy vegetables for your health

Salads for any occasion: salads can be much more than just a side dish

Home Vegetable Gardening: From Planning to Harvest, Learn How to Have Success

Healthy Shakes, Pies and Much More: Using Protein Drinks to Make Shakes and Pies and Other Healthy Ideas

Complete Guide to juicing for a healthy life

Enjoy!